Small Groups in Therapy Settings:

Process and Leadership

Small Groups in Therapy Settings:
Process and Leadership

Barbara W. Posthuma, M.Ed., OT (C)
Associate Professor
Department of Occupational Therapy
Faculty of Applied Health Sciences
University of Western Ontario
London, Ontario

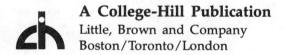

A College-Hill Publication
Little, Brown and Company
Boston/Toronto/London

College-Hill Press
A Division of
Little, Brown and Company (Inc.)
34 Beacon Street
Boston, Massachusetts 02108

Library of Congress Cataloging in Publication Data
Main entry under title:

Posthuma, Barbara W., 1931–
    Small groups in therapy settings : process and leadership / by
Barbara W. Posthuma.
        p.   cm.
    "A College-Hill publication."
    Bibliography: p.
    Includes index.
    ISBN 0-316-71474-7
    1. Occupational therapy.   2. Small groups.   3. Group relations
training.   I. Title.
RM735.P67   1989
616.89'1652 — dc 19   89-2808
                                                          CIP

ISBN 0-316-71474-7

Printed in the United States of America
           EB

To
Kristy and Kerry,
my original group

Contents

The road to wisdom? Well, it's plain
And simple to express:
Err
And err
And err again
But less
And less
And less

                              — Piet Hein

Preface

In spite of the fact that there are many books available on small groups, group process, and theories of groups, I have never been able to find the "right one" as a text for my course on group dynamics. This book grew out of that need, and it is my hope that it will fill a similar void for other educators. My methods of teaching the concepts of leadership and group dynamics are both didactic and experiential. I have attempted to write this text to reflect both these styles. Some chapters are minilectures, while others are conversational and echo past discussions with students. The latter style provoked a dilemma in the use of personal pronouns. Because most occupational therapists are female, I elected to use the female pronoun in all instances to refer to the leader-therapist and the male pronoun to refer to group members. This solution avoided using the awkward referent *he/she*.

Another dilemma was the use of the word "leader." It has been my experience that when students are learning to run therapeutic groups they tend to ignore (or are as yet unaware of) the therapeutic aspects and so they concentrate on "leading." Since I believe it is crucial for students to learn therapeutic leadership, I have, in an effort to reinforce this dual role, used the term *leader-therapist* in the conversational areas of the book. In the more general areas where the information is representative and pertinent to all types of group leaders I have used the single term, *leader*.

Students anticipate and look forward to actually working with clients and so their questions, for the most part, are very practical: "What should I do when . . . ?" or "What do you say . . . ?" In an effort to respond to these needs the content of the book leans heavily toward the clinical and applied aspects of interacting with clients in a therapeutic group. I have attempted to give concrete examples and suggestions of useful behaviors and responses to a variety of situations that leader-therapists are likely to encounter. From these suggestions I believe the learner can creatively expand and move on to trying her own ideas. I refer the reader to other texts for more theoretical information.

Whom is the book for? Although it was written from the perspective of an occupational therapist, I believe it has a broad appeal. Many facets of group dynamics and leadership are universal. Whether you are a nurse, a social worker, a psychologist, a counselor, or an occupational therapist (indeed, many work together in groups), you need the same basic information. Therefore, the general content of this book is thought to be appropriate for undergraduate students in other disciplines who are studying process and leadership of small groups. I also believe it can serve as a very useful reference and refresher text for clinicians working with groups or for those who are reentering the field.

Over many years of teaching group dynamics and leadership I have amassed much information from many sources, some known and some unknown, and it has gradually been rearranged into different forms for different purposes at different times. Through the passage of time, origins can be lost or displaced. If in the process of writing this text I have failed to credit an original source, it was certainly not intentional.

The information in the appendices is included to demonstrate how several group sessions can be organized around a single theme. The activities for each session are suggested and described to give the novice leader-therapist some format ideas as well as specific content ideas for immediate use.

I wish to acknowledge the help of several people in the preparation of the manuscript. First, I would like to thank Daniel Ling and Joyce McKinnon for facilitating the completion of the project. My appreciation also goes to colleagues Heather Emerson and Karen Harburn for reading sections of the book and offering comments, and to occupational therapists at Chedoke–McMaster Hospitals in Hamilton, Clarke Institute of Psychiatry in Toronto, Ottawa General Hospital, and Provincial Hospitals in Hamilton, Kingston, London, and St. Thomas for responding to my requests for activity and task ideas. I specifically thank the occupational therapists from Homewood Hospital in Guelph and Victoria Hospital in London for their information on assertiveness training. I offer my thanks to my colleagues for their understanding, to my students for their inspiration, to Rhonda Graves who enthusiastically did some of the drawings, to Jennifer Macnab for her calm responses to my cries for help with the computer, and especially to Anna Vandendries for assisting me in getting the book out of the computer. A special thanks goes to my daughter Kerry for the myriad ways in which she helped me throughout the production of the manuscript. My greatest debt of thanks goes to Allan, my partner in life, for his patience and tolerance while I did "the book."

B. W. P.

CHAPTER 1

The Small Group in Therapy

> *We must conclude that the psychology of groups is the oldest human psychology.*
> — SIGMUND FREUD

From the beginning of time people congregated in groups to ensure their own survival, development, and evolution. The knowledge that there was safety in numbers was a motivating factor in the earliest gatherings of people. Other factors that drew people together were spiritual in nature as groups of people congregated to worship, celebrate, and perform ritual dances. These original groups were formed naturally either by shared ancestry, mutual need, or common belief. In noting these beginnings Rudestam (1982) states: "Despite the pervasiveness of such groups throughout history, the connections between them and the deliberate use of group process to foster personality change in the twentieth century have not been made explicit" (p. 1). Although early theorists did not directly connect or address the behavior of individuals in groups in relation to therapeutic possibilities, sociologists and social psychologists did actively begin to raise questions and investigate the nuances of collective behavior late in the nineteenth century (Dunphy, 1972).

J. R. and L. M. Gibb (1978) observed that "groups form the fabric of the society in which we live" (p. 106) and early investigations were primarily focused on examining the effects of social influences on the behavior of individuals. One such exploration, credited to psychologist Normam Triplett in 1887, demonstrated that a cyclist's performance could be significantly improved if he was accompanied or paced by another rider (Bonner, 1959; Rudestam, 1982). Other researchers of this time studied the effect of working alone versus working in groups, pertaining to the performance of children in school, the influence of a group on thought processes, and the effect of competition on performance (Bonner, 1959). F. H. Allport, whose work is frequently documented in the early literature on groups, found that individuals working in a group produced more verbal associations and presented such associations with greater speed than did individuals working alone (Allport, 1920).

Later investigators (Comrey & Staats, 1955; Goldman, 1965) went on to compare individual and group performance using different combinations of individuals with varying initial ability. They found that the improved performance demonstrated by working in a dyad or a group was dependent on the initial ability levels of the individuals who were in combination.

In their review of the literature, Rosenbaum and Berger (1975) conclude that the primary early researchers noted for investigating small group phenomena were: Charles H. Cooley, who first defined the concept of "the primary group" as the "face to face" group primarily involved with "intimate cooperation"; Gustave Le Bon, who first described the group as a "collective entity — a distinct being"; and George Herbert Mead whose work, along with that of Cooley, was "of prime significance in the early history of group dynamics" (p. 13).

From these early explorations into the forces affecting individuals as they participated in groups evolved the use of groups as vehicles to promote change. One of the first practitioners credited with using this approach was Joseph Pratt, a Boston internist. Although Pratt originally used groups to save time in educating and supporting patients suffering from tuberculosis, he later became aware of the therapeutic value of the format, in particular the interactions among members of such groups. His work is acknowledged as an important forerunner to present-day psychotherapy (Rosenbaum, 1976; Rudestam, 1982).

Recognized as being the "founder of the study of modern group dynamics" (Luft, 1984, p. 8), social psychologist Kurt Lewin's work as a theorist and researcher in the investigation of group dynamics had a significant impact on the use of groups as agents for change (Smith, 1980a). The work of Lewin and his associates is credited with having a direct bearing on the invention of the T group (training group), from which evolved the encounter and sensitivity groups of the 1960s and 1970s. The widespread interest in these groups grew, in part, from the increased feelings of alienation that were experienced by an expanding portion of an increasingly mobile society (Ruitenbeek, 1970). Caring, trust, and the process of feedback, such as the sharing of perceptions both among members and with the leader, were encouraged in these groups. Emphasis was put on the importance of discussing events and behaviors happening in the "here-and-now" in the group.

Most reviews of the historical development of group work methods mark the advent of World War II as being a catalyst to increased interest and innovation in the use of groups (Lifton, 1972; Rosenbaum, 1976; Smith, 1980b; Rudestam, 1982). The shortage of trained therapists and the need to treat increasing numbers of disabled veterans precipitated a greater use of groups in therapy. Around this time the work of J. L. Moreno, who was "probably the most important individual in the history of group psychotherapy" (Shapiro, 1978, p. 22), was gaining much recognition. Today, Moreno is best remembered as the founder of psychodrama. In addition, he is credited with organizing the first society of group therapists coining the term "group psychotherapy" and introducing the first professional journal on group therapy (Rudestam, 1982). The basic premise of Moreno's psychodrama was an action technique to bring about both mental and emotional catharsis for the purpose of relieving tension. Although intense and extensive training is required today to qualify as a certified director of psychodrama, several of the individual techniques can be learned and effectively used by leader-therapists in small groups. Indeed, many explorative and spontaneous leader-therapists have intuitively used techniques such as role reversal and mirroring as part of role-playing sessions without thought of any connection to classic psychodrama.

Two trends emerged from 1932 to the mid-1960s in the years known as the "developmental period" of group psychotherapy (Shapiro, 1978). The first trend was the spreading application of the group method in the treatment of a wider variety of patient populations, and the second was the use of groups for purposes of personal growth and preservation. The latter trend produced an "explosion in numbers and kinds of groups" that began in the 1960s and has continued (Shapiro, 1978, p. 33). One would be remiss to leave even such a brief overview of the developmental period without noting the emergence of Alcoholics Anonymous. The founding of this movement in the late 1930s evolved from the awareness of the potency of individuals meeting together and interacting in a supportive way to produce change. This organization, which has a well-recorded success rate in helping alcoholics attain and maintain sobriety, is based on individuals coming together in groups for the shared experiences of disclosing, talking, listening, supporting, and learning (Alcoholics Anonymous World Service, 1984). Since then other self-help groups focusing on specific problem areas have evolved: Synanon, dealing with drug addiction; Al-Anon, a support group for family members of alcoholics; and more recently Tough-Love, a group formed by parents of children and adolescents who are troubled or in trouble.

ADVANTAGES OF GROUPS

Occupational therapists have brought patients together in one place for the purpose of being involved in activities since the inception of the profession. In the early years the activities that patients participated in under the official auspices of occupational therapy were primarily individual projects (Levine, 1987). At that time, when patients were organized collectively, the interactions that took place between them as they worked on their projects were not recognized or viewed as having particular therapeutic properties or significance (Howe & Schwartzberg, 1986). Gradually, since the mid-1930s, occupational therapists have gathered patients together into groups to participate in the unified experience of working together around a single project or activity. By the 1950s activity groups were found to enable clients to develop a feeling of belonging and an awareness of others, to increase socialization skills, to experience increased self-confidence, and to offer opportunities for the exchange of ideas (Nelson, Mackenthun, Bloesch, Milan, Unrein, & Hill, 1956). From the research and many investigations into all aspects of small groups that had been carried out by sociologists, psychologists, and psychiatrists, health professionals "recognized the group's curative powers and sought to use them to achieve therapeutic goals" (Howe & Schwartzberg, 1986, p. 52). Shannon and Snortum (1965) noted that "by working in a group of limited size, the patient could be provided with a more closely supervised opportunity for practicing rudimentary social skills and receive needed feedback from actual experience, thereby discovering that he is capable of handling social situations that formerly prompted his withdrawal" (p. 345).

Since then groups have proliferated with great vigor and variety among most of the helping professions. This very variety makes it difficult, and perhaps not wise, to generalize, but it seems safe to say that groups have been effective in short-term psychiatric settings (Bradlee, 1984; Prazoff, Joyce, & Azim, 1986; Youcha, 1976), long-term psychiatric settings (Waldinger, 1986; Wolf, 1975), and with the chronically physically ill (Buchanan, 1978; Levine, 1979). This expansion may, in part, be attributed to social psychologist Kurt Lewin who is credited with the observation that it is "usually easier to change individuals formed into a group than to change any one of them separately" (Rosenbaum & Berger, 1975, p. 16).

THE THERAPEUTIC GROUP

The main purpose of all therapeutic endeavors is to bring about change. When an occupational therapist involves a patient in a sanding project a probable goal is to increase muscle strength or range of motion or both (Pedretti, 1985).

When a patient is given the antipsychotic drug chlorpromazine it is often to alleviate the symptoms of acute psychosis (Waldinger, 1986). In a therapeutic small group the specific goals for each member can be varied but would include the expectation that change will occur (Levine, 1979).

Often groups are called by names that indicate their purpose. For example, therapists run communication groups, assertiveness groups, life skills groups, and decision making groups. The general goals of these respective groups would be to improve communication skills, to increase assertiveness, to provide experience in life skills, and to allow experience in a decision making process.

If the theme of the group is self-awareness, then one goal for the group members would be to become more aware of various aspects of themselves — how they behave in different situations, how they react to certain stimuli, and how others react and behave in return. A second goal would be for the members to use this new awareness in gaining a better understanding of themselves and, based on this understanding, to effect some change in their behavior directed at achieving or eliciting more productive outcomes.

Immediately the question arises, "What happens in groups that enables members to change?" Or as Kottler (1983) asks, "What is this magic that cures people of their suffering?" (p. 51). In commenting on the process and the helpful aspects of therapeutic groups, Ellis (1974) describes one benefit as removing the "magic" quality from therapy by emphasizing the need for "persistent hard work" (p. 109). Although a patient does not experience the same one-to-one attention in a group that he would receive during individual therapy there are other factors that contribute to the success of groups as a therapeutic modality. Rudestam (1982) discusses five elements that he considers to be advantages for using groups in therapy.

He likens a group to a "miniature society" where members can lose their feelings of alienation and, temporarily at least, experience feelings of belonging, thus meeting one of the basic needs of mankind (Maslow, 1962). Within the group setting members can experience everyday life situations such as peer pressure, social influence, and the need to conform. When these experiences occur in a learning environment, such as a group, then the changes that occur are usually transferable to the outside world (Rudestam, 1982; Posthuma, 1972).

The second element in favor of the group treatment setting is the opportunity to be among others with whom common problems can be shared. It offers the chance to learn new skills and behaviors in a supportive environment. Through group interaction one can receive feedback and caring, experience trust and acceptance, and learn new ways of relating to others. Since most groups are comprised of a cross section of members of society at large, this affords each group member opportunities to cope with give-and-take situations similar to those existing in the world outside. In one-to-one therapy the client experiences only one other point of view and one source of feedback, that of the therapist. While such viewpoints and feedback may be valid, they are limited in breadth and experience by virtue of coming from only one person (Ellis, 1974). In a group the client may experience several points of view and varied feedback, as shown in Figure 1-1, all of which may be presented in different ways. It is with and from this assortment of information that the group

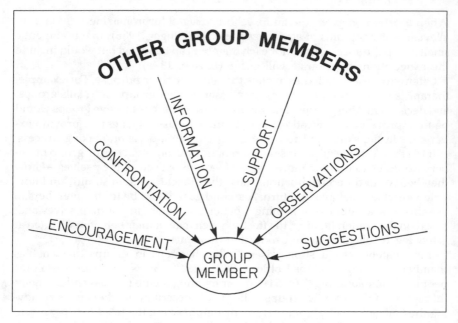

Figure 1-1. Sample of varied feedback available to each group member.

member is able to sort through and select. Hopefully, because of this mixture, he will get a broader view of himself and become more aware of the more subtle nuances in his behavior. Also, the integration of information is likely to produce a combination of supportive and confrontive messages which can soften any good-bad or right-wrong dichotomies. The more supportive feedback serves as a sort of cushion for the more confrontive. In essence this multifeedback situation creates an environment in which members are more receptive and would feel less need to be defensive and block out negative feedback (Hansen, Warner, & Smith, 1976). They are more apt to listen, to take in and consider what they hear, and hence benefit from the process. Conversely, it is also true that there is strength in numbers. It is easier to disregard feedback that comes from one source only with a what-does-he-know? attitude. However, it is close to impossible to ignore feedback from five or more persons if they share the same perceptions and are all giving you the same messages or information.

Third, the individual is able to observe the problems, struggles, behaviors, interaction styles, and coping mechanisms of the others in the group. He is then able to use this information as a yardstick for comparing his own behaviors. From this he can assess his own abilities and disabilities and consider possibilities for personal change.

Closely linked to the third advantage is the fourth, which is the facilitation of the individual growth process. The support of the group can be an enhancing factor in self-exploration and introspection (Posthuma & Posthuma, 1972).

Feeling, caring, and respect from others can go a long way in promoting the self-confidence necessary to attempt new and different ways of behaving.

The final advantage of the group format for therapy noted by Rudestam (1982) is the obvious one of economics. Having several patients meet together with a leader-therapist rather than meeting individually with the therapist saves time and money.

TERMINOLOGY

Before going further a clarification of terminology is in order. In any discussion of small groups the terms *group dynamics* and *group process* are frequently used. Comments such as "There were some powerful dynamics in that group" or "The process in the group today was really interesting" are often made by leader-therapists or observers of small group sessions. So what do these terms mean? While noting that the term group dynamics can refer to a field of study and a body of knowledge, Knowles and Knowles (1972) define group dynamics in its most basic sense as "the complex forces that are acting upon every group throughout its existence which cause it to behave the way it does" (p. 14). The term group process, Fried (1972) says, should be used specifically to refer to the patterns of interactions that develop among members at various times during a group. However, because the complex forces and the interactions are all occurring simultaneously it can be seen that the forces may well affect the interactions, and conversely, the interactions among the members may alter and affect the forces. Because of this concurrent, intimate, and ongoing relationship between the two, for the purposes of this book the two terms will be used interchangeably to mean the same thing: everything and anything that is happening in a group, whether the occurrence is seen to be overt or covert.

HOW CHANGE OCCURS

Change leads people into the realm of the unknown and the realization of this can be frightening (Thompson & Kahn, 1970). There are no certainties with change, and undefined future experiences and situations create resistance to change in everyone. People invest a great deal of energy in preserving the status quo as a defense against change. People often say "that's the way I am" as a means of ending any further discussion of behaviors or alternatives.

There are no guarantees that change will make things better for a person or that significant others will agree on what constitutes "better." When a person does change some aspect of his way of "being" in the world, the change in his behavior will not necessarily be seen as beneficial by all who are close to him (Posthuma & Posthuma, 1973). For example, a woman who finds herself with the multiple roles of wife, mother, homemaker, and secretary may suddenly feel overwhelmed by this load and decide that some of the family responsibilities should be assumed by her husband. Her husband, satisfied with things the way they are, may not react positively to this change from passive to assertive behavior on the part of his wife and thus may resist her demands. If the husband refuses to change his ways his wife will not only continue to feel overwhelmed but will probably feel angry as well. If the husband agrees to help and assumes some of what he sees as his wife's responsibilities he may then feel resentful and angry. The conflicts arising from such a situation obviously need to be resolved, through compromise or other solutions, to enable the couple to proceed with their lives together in harmony.

The need for change comes when people find some aspect of their lives unbearable, or when those close to them find aspects of their behavior unacceptable (Hansen, Warner, & Smith, 1976). Factors such as loneliness, a poor relationship, lack of a job, drinking, fears, or losses may be experienced as problems. Kanfer and Goldstein (1986) state that generally psychological problems are related to difficulties in relationships, in attitudes toward the self or in the perceptions of the environment. They cite four characteristics (presented here in part) that they believe indicate evidence of the presence of a psychological problem.

1. The person experiences discomfort, worry, or fears that are not easily remedied by some action that he can perform without assistance.
2. The person shows a behavioral deficiency or excessively engages in some behavior that is assessed by himself or others to interfere with his functioning.
3. The person engages in activities that are objectionable to those around him and that lead to negative consequences either for himself or for others.
4. The person shows behavioral deviations that result in severe social sanctions by those in the immediate environment (p. 8).

The beginning of the change process is marked by the recognition that something must be altered. At this point the individual may try to make changes by himself, or he may turn to family members or friends. He may seek out a counselor or therapist or join a therapeutic group. Whatever avenue he chooses through which to find help, the change process that ensues tends to be similar. In relationship with others he finds individuals, therapists, or group members who accept him and listen to his thoughts and feelings. Within this environment of acceptance and positive regard he is able to recognize and realize the existence of previously denied feelings and behaviors (Rogers, 1951). This enables the client to reorganize his self-perceptions in ways that allow him to gradually accept himself and see himself as a person of worth who is worthy of becoming even more.

Yalom (1970) discusses "curative factors" that he says operate in all types of therapy groups, with different factors being emphasized in any given group depending on the goals and composition of the group and the approach that is being used. It is also true that in some situations clients must deal with certain factors before they can benefit from others (Bonney, Randall, & Cleveland, 1986). Yalom notes that many of the factors are interdependent and that some factors represent conditions for change while others are actually mechanisms of change. Yalom's factors have been extensively cited and investigated, including recent research that explored the timing of testing as being a determinant of which factors group members would consider to be the most effective change agents. MacKenzie (1987) established that outcome measures retrospectively evaluating the usefulness of the curative factors differed from results obtained while members were still active in the group.

The ten primary categories of the curative factors are as follows (Yalom, 1970, pp. 5–14):

1. *Imparting of Information.* The type of information imparted in groups will depend on the type of group, the leader, and the members. Included may be advice, suggestions, guidance, interpretations, or didactic instruction about a certain theoretical approach such as transactional analysis or cognitive restructuring. In occupational therapy the instructions to a group may be given in areas such as assertive behavior, life skills, or goal setting. One must be careful in using a didactic approach that the group does not become essentially a "class" and hence foster a dependence on the leader to "tell us what to do." This caution is basically supported by the work of Block and Crouch (1985) who found "guidance" to be one of the least helpful curative factors.

2. *Installation of Hope.* It is crucial that members see the group as a helpful-hopeful treatment method. Most occupational therapy groups are open, so new members are being accepted as others approach discharge. This process offers the opportunity for those members who have gained and improved from the group experience to share their experiences with the newer members. If Joe can say, "When I first came into this group I was scared and didn't think I had anything worthwhile to say, so I was pretty quiet. But now I think I talk as much as anyone," then this can give encouragement and hope to a timid, withdrawn member that he too may be able to reach that point. Yalom (1970) actually encourages leaders to "exploit" this factor by pointing out changes and improvements that members have made as a means of offering hope to others.

3. *Universality.* Each group member is different, having his very own set of unique problems. Members often believe that no one else could possibly have problems that are as bad as theirs. However, as members begin to talk in the group and as the "bad" problems are shared, members come to experience a join-the-club feeling. As members listen to disclosures made by other clients they sense a similarity of concerns and issues. This helps them put their own problems into perspective and tends to alleviate their feelings of aloneness which dissolves the feeling of "I am the only one." In a study of three self-help groups, Lieberman (1983) reports that universality, the feeling of being with others who share the same problems, was the experience that the members valued the most. In losing their feelings of uniqueness members came to perceive their thoughts and feelings not as being aberrant and unusual but as being

quite common among those with similar problems. While this dispelling of feelings of isolation is therapeutic in itself, it also facilitates a feeling of unity among the members that is the very foundation for a successful group.

4. *Altruism.* One of the basic premises of therapeutic groups is that the members will help each other. The trust and cohesion that evolve in groups supply fertile ground for patients to give feedback, reassurance, suggestions, and support to one another. Since many patients who are members of therapy groups suffer from low self-esteem, this process of being able to help others can be a very ego-strengthening experience. It is often the group members, rather than the leader-therapist, who offer caring and point out one another's strengths and assets.

5. *Family Reenactment.* Although other researchers (Block, Crouch, & Reibstein, 1981; MacDevitt & Sanislow, 1987) have found family reenactment to be one of the least helpful curative factors, Yalom (1970) recognized the familial aspects of a therapeutic group as being useful. Many patients will have had unsatisfactory, if not traumatic, family experiences. Reporting on a study involving a group of incest victims, Bonney, Randall, and Cleveland (1986) found that the members placed a heavy emphasis on gaining genetic insight through self-understanding and family reenactment. As well as gaining understanding of the past, being in a therapy group gives members the opportunity to experience what can be felt as a caring family environment. Within this group "family" they can discuss and perhaps resolve issues from their primary family such as parent-child conflicts and sibling rivalries. Borrowing from their professional colleagues the psychodramatists, occupational therapists often use role playing in their groups to re-create family situations in order that members can learn new ways of relating and interacting within their own families.

6. *Development of Socializing Techniques.* The assessment and development of social skills has long been of prime interest to occupational therapists. Social skills are prerequisites for most people to function adequately in their life roles. However, most of our patients experience difficulties in one if not several of their life roles and their problems can, in part, be based on poor social skills. The process of feedback, mentioned earlier, affords the opportunity to learn about one's maladaptive social behavior. For patients who lack close personal relationships in their lives the group is often the first time they have had the opportunity to give and receive personal feedback. Role playing, a technique often used in groups, can be used successfully both in increasing awareness of and in teaching social skills. This technique is discussed more fully in Chapter 13.

7. *Imitative Behavior.* In any group each participant has the opportunity to observe at close hand and in an interactive manner, the behaviors of all the other participants. Through such observations, they become aware of which behaviors evoke positive and negative responses from the other members. By imitating or "trying on" these behaviors they too can evoke such responses. Behaviors that receive a positive reaction from others are usually repeated and hence new learning can occur. Some members may imitate certain behaviors of the leaders or other members only to later discard them, deciding the "fit" is not comfortable. This too is learning. Of course there can also be the member who

imitates the "bad" person in the group in order to receive the same degree of attention, even if it is negative attention.

8. *Interpersonal Learning.* No one goes through life alone. Rudestam (1982) says, "Life is primarily a social event" (p. 6). A person may feel lonely and alienated or be considered a loner but the demands of daily existence, be they work or play, tend to involve one in relating to others. Because a group is considered a social microcosm (Yalom, 1983) or miniature society (Rudestam, 1982) it presents similar demands. Initially, members of a group, or a new member in an ongoing group, may monitor and control how they behave. However, it is anticipated that eventually each person will relax and come to behave as he normally does in his own social environment. He will affect the other members of the group in much the same way as he affects people with whom he has contact in the greater society. By virtue of the purpose and the process of a therapeutic group, members will receive feedback on their "way of being" and from these reactions and responses they have the opportunity to learn how they affect others. Spurred by this feedback, and the support and encouragement of the group, they can, it is hoped, go on to learning more productive ways of interacting. The trust and caring that develops in a group creates a safer environment for experimentation and trying out new ways of relating than the environment of society at large.

In an assessment of Yalom's curative factors Lewis (1987) states a case for the importance of interactions between people in the process of bringing about change. He believes that a person can interact with another in a way to elicit a desired response. He refers to these as "complementary responses" and because they are new and different from the person's usual response style they constitute a change. Positive reactions to the new interactive style serve as a reward and reinforcer for continuance of the changed behavior. Lewis's point is in keeping with the belief that people often live up (or down) to perceived expectations.

9. *Cohesion.* The concept of cohesion is central to any discussion of the elements contributing to the successful functioning of groups. The concept has been accorded many definitions but they all have a common theme (Brilhart, 1974). Words such as "unity," "bonded," "we-ness," "cemented," and "loyalty" are all used to describe a state of cohesion in a group. Lewin (1947) described cohesiveness as the "total field of forces which act on members to remain in the group" (p. 30). Yalom (1970) also notes that it is not a static state, but rather that the degree of cohesiveness present in a group fluctuates over time and circumstance. He goes on to point out that cohesion in and of itself does not have therapeutic properties but is an important determinant of effective therapy occurring. It is during periods when a group is experiencing a feeling of unity or togetherness that members are more apt to contribute, take risks, interact, and be productive (Penland & Fine, 1974). Members who are attracted to the group, feel accepted, and experience a sense of belonging are more apt to express and explore themselves, relate more meaningfully, be more tolerant of conflict, and attend regularly (Dimock, 1985a). In terms of group process, Lakin (1983) sees cohesiveness among group members as giving them an emotional investment in the task and in one another, prompting greater stability in the presence of frustration, and allowing a diversity in the members' aims and goals.

10. *Catharsis.* Catharsis refers to the expression of strong emotions and usually emotions that have not been previously expressed (Loomis, 1979). Although this curative factor was described as "low prestige but irrepressible" by Yalom (p. 71) in 1970, in later research it emerged as being the most important factor (Long & Cope, 1980). By 1985 Yalom found catharsis to be one of the four factors valued most highly by a variety of outpatients in eight different investigations. In the perspective of today's highly pressured society this high ranking can be seen to make a lot of sense. Many of us live our lives by controlling our emotions and not showing the world how we really feel. To display emotions, especially in public, is generally considered poor form and a sign of weakness. Indeed, boys especially are frequently admonished to hide their feelings and "be a big boy" or "be a man." Therefore it is not surprising that when these restrictions and attitudes are not present, as in a group, that individuals experience a sense of freedom and release from tension. These good feelings come from being allowed and even encouraged to "get it off our chest" while still feeling respect and acceptance.

Moreno (1957) spoke of the healing effect of catharsis and Janov (1972) of expunging "primal" pain through catharsis. A study by Lieberman, Yalom, and Miles (1973) pointed out that catharsis per se was not necessarily curative, but when coupled with a form of cognitive learning it could produce a positive outcome. Behaviors that are considered to be cathartic in nature and therapeutic in outcome are the expression of feelings about the self or the expression of positive or negative feelings to others. Such expressions need not always be intense or explosive to be cathartic. The act of a group member mildly expressing how he is feeling can be a new and freeing event for that individual and can frequently evoke similar output from others.

Yalom's ten curative factors endorse the belief that groups are a valuable modality in facilitating change. The need for change is often precipitated by one of the many transitions that people face in a society of "temporary structure" (Seashore, 1974). Temporariness is evident in the high divorce rate, increased geographic relocations, broken families, career changes, and shortened careers. Some persons manage to adjust and functionally survive the stresses in their lives, while others, unable to cope, retreat with their problems into a world of varying degrees of dysfunction. Groups have been experienced and found to be of significance by both types of persons. For those who are adapting and adjusting, groups have served to enhance their coping skills. For the others, groups are therapeutic in nature and remedial in intent (Smith, Wood, & Smale, 1980). While all therapeutic groups are oriented to change, some focus primarily on intrapsychic and intrapersonal change, whereas others focus on effecting change in interpersonal skills and relationships.

SUMMARY

The concept of people living and working together is as old as time itself. Although various congregations of people may have been at war or in conflict with each other the individuals within each group were held together by common purposes and feelings of safety and belonging.

Similar basic aspects pull people together today. People join groups because they like the others in the group, they like the activity or purpose of the group, they want to experience feelings of belonging, or they find they can only accomplish a personal goal by joining with others (e.g., to be a leader, help a cause, or participate in an activity). It can be useful for leaders of therapeutic groups to keep these basic motives in mind when organizing and trying to meet the needs of the members in their groups.

Participating in a group can be a powerful social experience, as it can be motivating, enlightening, and emotional. As various professionals noted these social effects on individuals who were involved in groups, the professionals became more and more aware of the significance of group interaction. Generally, groups have come to be seen as valuable because they allow members opportunities to have the following positive experiences:

1. A sense of belonging
2. Sharing common problems
3. Observing behaviors and consequences of behaviors in others
4. Support during self-exploration and change

Therapeutically, groups are useful because they bring people together to work on their individual problems in concert. The curative factors that occur when individuals are in interaction are:

1. Sharing information
2. Gaining hope
3. Sharing problems
4. Helping one another
5. Experiencing the group as a family
6. Developing social skills
7. Imitating behaviors of others
8. Learning and trying out new behaviors
9. Experiencing cohesion with others
10. Expressing emotions

Groups have great therapeutic value for persons with minor or severe problems, with or without insight, and in formal or informal settings. Using groups in therapy can also solve certain economic problems, as several persons can work together at the same time with one therapist.

CHAPTER 2

Group Development

*I am not now that which I
have been.*

— LORD BYRON

Before the meaning of a group's developmental process can be grasped it is necessary to understand the structure of groups and how a group is conceptualized in the overall scheme of things. The perspective chosen from which to examine a group is that of the group as a system. It is hoped that the following brief discussion of a group from this framework will emphasize the many intricacies and complexities inherent in any group. Having established a group as a many-faceted entity, the rest of the chapter will be given to the presentation of two models of group development.

Discrepancies existed among the pioneering researchers in how they viewed and described the phenomenon called a group. There were those who believed that a group was the sum of its parts: a collective of individual persons participating together. In other words, even though the persons were participating in a group, they in essence remained individuals and did not form a whole (Bonner, 1959).

Others believed that although a group was a collection of individuals, their individuality was affected by virtue of the act that they had come together as a group. By coming together, the group of individuals was no longer the sum of its parts, but was a complete entity in and of itself.

Having presented these opposing views, Bonner then went on to observe that neither one was accurate. He argued that an individual member in a group did not remain as such, but entered into a mutual relationship with others in the group. Because of this mutuality he did not see the group as an entity unto itself, but rather noted that the group presented a pattern of interacting persons. Thus Bonner concluded that a group was a *network of psychological relationships*. This network will now be examined.

THE GROUP AS A SYSTEM

Closely related to Bonner's conclusion is the definition of a system set forth by Hall and Fagen (1968). They state: "A system is a set of *objects* together with *relationships* between the objects and between their *attributes* (p. 81) (italics added). Hall and Fagen go on to explain that the *objects* of a system are considered to be the "parts or components" which are "unlimited in variety." The *attributes* are described as the "properties of the objects" and the *relationships* are what "tie the system together." A system, then, is made up of a variety of parts each of which also has properties and all of which are tied together by relationships.

Applying Hall and Fagen's definition to a group, the following identifications can be made. The "parts" are perceived as the group members, the "properties" as the personalities of the members, and the "relationships" as the feelings and interactions, both verbal and nonverbal, that occur among the members. In other words, a small group is conceived to be a system (Watzlawick, Beavin, & Jackson, 1967).

To be more specific, it is believed that a small group represents an *open system* (Barker, Wahlers, Cegala, & Kibler, 1983) since it does not always maintain a steady state but is constantly developing and moving toward a steady state or homeostasis (Bertalanffy, 1968). This phenomenon of homeostasis is a useful concept to understand and to apply in the observation of the workings of a small group. It presupposes that the "individual," be it atom, cell, animal, or man, interacts with its environment and is governed by certain principles of equilibrium or homeostasis (Hall & Fagen, 1968). The individual has a preferred state of homeostasis and will consistently behave in a manner to maintain such a state. As the individual experiences his environment by behaving in certain ways, and experiences the behavior of others toward him, this state of equilibrium may be altered. Because of feelings of discomfort with this altered state and the need to return to the preferred state of equilibrium, the individual will behave in ways to try to bring this about.

The same phenomenon occurs in a group. The group as an entity itself can be thought to desire a state of homeostasis. When any behavioral change occurs in a group member it affects every other member and hence the group as a whole (Steiner, 1972; Palazzolo, 1981). This precipitates reactionary behaviors in the other members in an attempt to regain a state of equilibrium or homeostasis (Heap, 1977). For example, this process might be diagrammed as in Figure 2-1. Here, the group is depicted initially in a comfortable state and then when a group member says, "I'm feeling very sad," the other members immediately become activated to deal with the situation. They may try to explore with the member why he is feeling sad and they will almost surely offer advice on what he could or should do to overcome his sadness. A member is then most likely to ask a question such as, "Has this discussion helped?," or "Are you feeling any

Figure 2-1. Maintenance of homeostasis among group members.

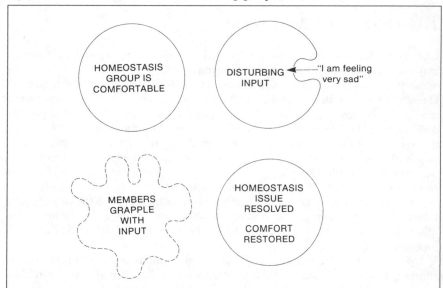

better now?," which demonstrates the group's need to feel that the member is no longer sad and that they, including the distressed member, have returned to a state of equilibrium. One can usually tell when this state has been reached, as the group members appear to relax. You may even see an actual relaxing of body postures: members usually become quiet, even physically still, and seem to be in a rather tranquil state.

This desire for a preferred state of comfort or balance can also be observed in the situation where the group appears to be comfortable but suddenly a member says something like, "I'm still upset by what John said about Mary." An interjection such as this will usually mobilize the group instantly. Members immediately query not only the member who made the statement but also Mary, to determine if she is upset and John to find out if he intended to be "upsetting." Through this process the members are really saying that they feel uncomfortable with this state of disequilibrium and they want to "fix" it so they can return to a more comfortable state. Not only may the presence of negative feelings cause members to react, but any intense situation, such as the sharing of intimate feelings or a deep emotional reaction, can elicit feelings of discomfort or embarrassment. Members then make efforts to regain a sense of balance in the emotional climate, as depicted in Figure 2-2, which is often attempted through an abrupt change of topic or focus. This need for a steady state can be

Figure 2-2. Members attempting to regain emotional balance.

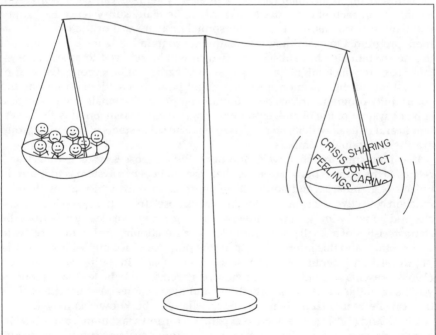

likened metaphorically to a jellyfish or even a drop of mercury. If you nudge either one of them they will move or roll around until they have accommodated the effect of the nudge and have once again attained what is for them a state of homeostasis.

The process just described encompasses the three perspectives from which Rapoport (1968) observes both living and nonliving systems. These fundamental aspects are structure, function, and evolution, or in terms more relative to a group's desire for equilibrium, being, action, and becoming. Looking again at Figure 2-2 the group can initially be seen to be in a state of "being." An "action" occurs, "I'm feeling very sad," which throws the group into the process of "becoming." No matter how the group functions at this stage it will eventually regain a state of being, although this state will not be the same as before, as the group will have evolved to a new or different way of being, (not necessarily better, only different).

In examining the world with all its complexities, it can be seen to be either one mammoth system or it can be seen as being made up of an infinite number of smaller systems. Hence some systems can be parts of a larger whole and can be called *subsystems* (Hall & Fagen, 1968)

Now let us think in more practical and relevant terms. For example, consider an entity that most occupational therapists have had some experience with: a general hospital. The whole hospital may be regarded as a system, but it can also be thought of as comprising or encompassing many subsystems. Each department in the hospital can be seen as a system, as can each ward. And again, within each of these there are likely to be many subsystems. Each ward will have subsystems, such as the personnel on that ward or the overall treatment program. On examining the treatment program in Figure 2-3 we see that this subsystem also has subsystems (which will be referred to as sub-subsystems), one of which might be known as a small group or task group. Other sub-subsystems of the treatment program might be the recreational program, the community program, or the chemotherapy program. The small group may be a sub-subsystem of the overall treatment program subsystem, but it is also a system in and of itself with its own subsystems. The subsystems of the small group are the individual members.

It is interesting to note how Kielhofner (1985) discusses systems theory as it relates to the human body. He states that "the concept of a system is that certain objects (e.g., muscles and bones) have interrelationships which allow them to function collectively toward an identifiable purpose" (p. 2). If one replaces "muscles and bones" with "group members," then the statement clearly describes the characteristics of a small group. Members of a functioning group must relate to one another, and this interrelating is for the purpose of accomplishing or working toward an "identifiable purpose" or a *group goal*. In earlier work, Jordon (1968) presents a broad and open view of systems. He believes that as long as you have entities that can be identified and connections between the entities that can be recognized, then you have what can be known as a system.

Checkland (1981) sees a need to expand on Jordon's taxonomy, and presents a more precise and detailed approach to defining systems by differentiating

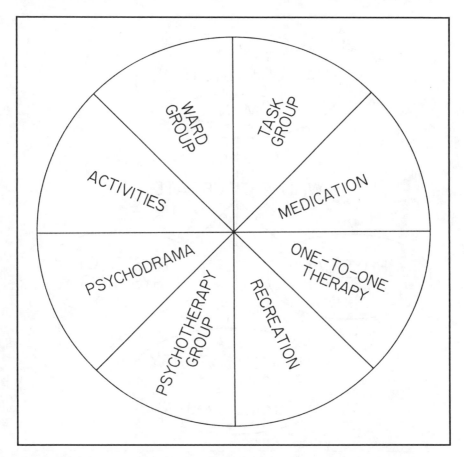

Figure 2-3. Subsystems of the treatment program.

four classes of systems as shown in Figure 2-4: (1) natural systems, (2) designed physical systems, (3) designed abstract systems, and (4) human activity systems. To see how the small group fits into this overall classification a brief comment on each type of system is included here.

1. *Natural Systems.* These are physical systems that began at the origin of the universe. Their form was determined by the forces, processes, and evolution going on at that time, and their characteristics will remain the same as long as these determining factors remain the same. Thus the physical framework of the earth and other planets is considered to be a natural system. For example, the sun always rises in the east and sets in the west. The natural system of most relevance to our discussion is that of the human being: the individual person.

2. *Designed Physical Systems.* Such systems differ from natural systems in that they can be altered; they are the result of what man has made by conscious

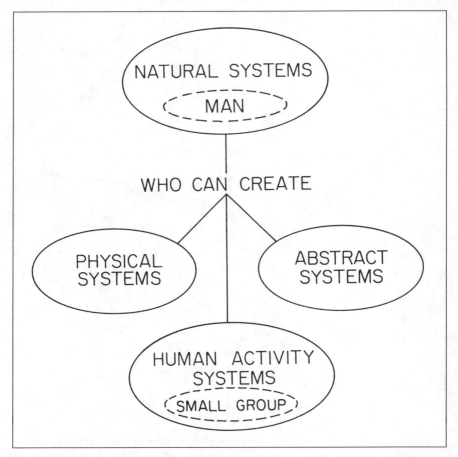

Figure 2-4. Four classes of systems. (Source: Modified from P. Checkland. *Systems thinking, systems practice.* New York: Wiley, 1981.)

design. They came about due to a need within man or a need perceived by man, and so the point of their being is to serve a purpose. The telephone system designed by man is a perfect example; it is one way to meet man's desire for communication and, even at times, the need to survive. A concrete object like a book is also said to be a designed physical system, and has the purpose of preserving and disseminating information.

3. *Designed Abstract Systems.* If we look back to the previous example given to describe a designed physical system, that is, a book, it will lead us to an understanding of designed abstract systems. Being without physical properties, these systems evolve as conscious thoughts and ideas from man's mind and are the stuff from which books, records, and films are made. Like the physical sys-

tems, they too serve a purpose, which might be the expansion of knowledge or the expression of the creative side of humans.

4. *Human Activity Systems.* This class of systems is the largest of the four and the one to which our entity of interest, a small group, belongs. While these systems are not as tangible as the natural and designed systems, they are obvious entities with an underlying purpose. They consist of a number of activities related in a manner that gives the whole relevancy. In the case of the small group, the activities will be those of each group member as he relates to the productivity of the group and its goals. Although the small group is made up of human beings, which are themselves natural systems, the group as an entity is considered to be a human activity system: alternatively, a *system of systems.*

It is this concept of a whole and its parts, a system of systems, that is of importance to those who lead or are involved in small groups. Leader-therapists must always be aware that their group is made up of several members, each of whom has his or her own individuality, expressed or not expressed as needs, wishes, fears, or caring. Although these members or subsystems, when together, do form a whole or system (i.e., the group), it is very important to constantly be aware of and sensitive to their functioning as individuals. It can be difficult for a leader-therapist to do this consistently.

Take for example a group where the goal or task for a given session is to rank-order a list of attributes by the process of consensus. As the group begins there is a lively discussion by most members, and it can be easy for the leader-therapist to get caught up in the content or productivity of the large system while ignoring one or more of the subsystems (individual members). It may appear as if the group or large system is functioning very well as it moves quickly and perhaps efficiently toward the completion of the task. On close observation of the individuals, however, it might be the case that one member is not participating at all.

It can be easy to miss such an occurrence if the leader-therapist is focusing almost exclusively on the larger system. She needs to be aware of all the subsystems, sensitive to their individuality and to their unique needs and ways of functioning and expressing themselves. Since each individual has input into the group (even lack of input is input), the total system will be affected. These initial and ongoing actions and interactions meld into a process that can be observed and compartmentalized as the group develops.

THE PROCESS OF GROUP DEVELOPMENT

Similar to the way in which Eric Erikson (1963) set out his theory of stages of development in a person, theorists have described developmental stages for groups. We refer to a group as having a life of its own and just as each human life is different from others so is each group, and each session of any specified group, different from others. A group is not a static thing but rather it ebbs and flows in different ways and at different paces. Just as a person's development can be arrested at a certain stage, so too can a group plateau for a time at a certain stage or regress to an earlier stage. The question is whether there is any consistent form to the changes that occur in groups. Are there definitive stages that a group passes through on its way to becoming a functioning unit, and do all groups move through the same stages? The answer is that all groups do experience different stages although the boundaries are vague at times and groups may function in overlapping stages.

THE AUTHORITY CYCLE

This perspective presents the stages of group development in terms of the relationship between the leader and group members. It describes the feelings, behavior and movement of group members as being directly related to the behavior of the leader. At the beginning of the cycle or development of the group, authority is seen as being invested in the leader. As the group develops, this authority is gradually transferred from the leader to the members. This is not always a smooth passage, and as can be seen in Figure 2-5 there are several stages.

The first stage of the authority cycle is that of *dependence* (A). This is the starting point of most groups and at this point the members are dependent on the leader for direction and total support. There is little if any interaction between members as they look to the leader to tell them what to do and explain what is expected of them. Gemmill (1986) uses the term "deskill" to describe how group members embrace what he refers to as the "leader-myth," by denying their own abilities and resources to perform and function independently as a

Figure 2-5. Stages of the authority cycle.

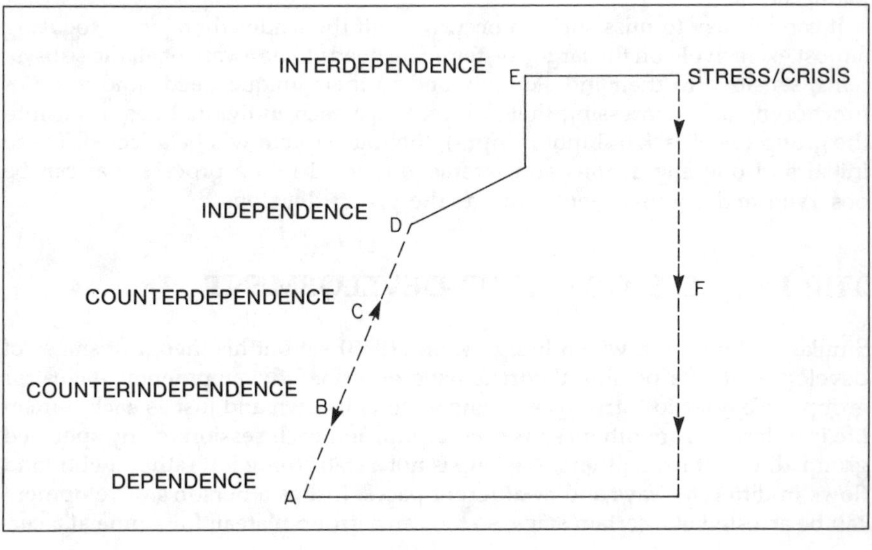

group. He portrays the members as projecting all their coping and creative skills onto the designated leader. By deskilling themselves the members strengthen the authority of the leader and reinforce their own feelings of confusion, helplessness, and dependency. As the leader tries to move out of this authoritative role by offering the group its freedom (freedom of choice, freedom to decide, freedom to make the group their own), the group's initial reaction is often one of hostility. Members prefer a comfortable structural situation where they are told what to do over one where they experience the insecurity of having to accept responsibility. This stage is known as the *counterindependence* stage (B) and the general feeling in the group is one of fear and anger. Members are hostile to the leader because he is not living up to their expectations of him. He is not telling them what to do, organizing or doing things for them. Generally, in their eyes he is not being a "good leader."

When the group finally accepts the fact that it has some freedom to make decisions and determine its own life, it begins to move away from the leader, and this stage is known as *counterdependence* (C). This stage is often characterized by a struggle for leadership among the members. As the members realize that the established leader is not going to do the job, group members begin to assert themselves by vying for the role. This movement away from the leader is often accompanied by expressions of hostility ("All right, if you aren't going to do the job we'll show you"), or rejection ("We can get along without you"). At this point the group tries to establish some norms and patterns of operation which will provide the stability it needs to function independently of the leader. If the leader does not grant the group freedom to express its hostility, the group may stifle its anger, become resistive, and group growth may be inhibited. The leader must be willing to suffer the discomfort of some rejection and hostility in order to help the group progress to accepting responsibility for itself. This stage is usually one of tension and strain. The group therefore is not very creative and morale may be low.

If the leader accepts the group's declaration of independence displayed in the counterdependence stage, the group is free to enter a new phase of its existence which is known as the stage of *independence* (D). This stage is usually a joyful one for the group. As they experience their freedom and independence they may take flight from reality through laughter and giddiness. The leader may experience a feeling of being left out as the general attitude of the members is one of ignoring the leader. Members frequently behave in ways that convey, "See, we don't need you; we can do this by ourselves." Frequently at this stage, members resist getting on with the business of the group as they enjoy their independence, the heightened morale of the group, and their new feelings of togetherness. The group begins to feel strong as a unit and as a result of this members display increased confidence and comfort.

As these feelings of confidence and unity among the members strengthen, the members stop fighting the leader and permit the leader to reenter the group. This is done by listening to and accepting any contributions now made by the leader. Since the group experiences a sense of control over what is happening, this feeling is extended to allow the leader to participate. This sense of control that members feel also allows them to feel safe in their relationships with one another and paves the way for the group to move on to the *interdependence* stage (E). At this stage members interact in equal, encouraging, and supportive ways with one another and with the leader.

As long as there are no undue events or pressures on the group it may continue to function very productively and creatively at this stage of interdependence. However, should a crisis or something untoward occur, then the group may fall back (F) to the stage of dependence (A) with a "How do we handle this?," or "What do we do now?" approach to the leader. Rosenbaum and Rosenbaum (1971) cite examples of subjects, on encountering obstacles or difficult tasks, reverting to dependency by seeking direction. The leader's response to such an occurrence is crucial to the continued functional health of the group. A leader may intentionally or unintentionally welcome the dependence and move to actively take over the group again by telling them to "do this" or "do that." If the leader follows this with further controlling behavior she will find the group entrenched again at the dependence stage, in effect back at square one. However, the leader who responds to the crisis event at the interdependent stage with a problem solving approach enables the group to maintain its interdependent functional abilities. Rather than telling the members what they should do the leader-therapist might ask, "What do you think we should do?," "What alternatives do we have?," or "What might help?" By engaging with the members in this problem solving approach the leader is emphasizing the interdependence of members with one another and with the leader. She is also giving the members a message of faith in their functional abilities: a message that says, "I'll help, but I also need your help and together we can work this out."

If a group does revert back to an earlier stage of development, it is usually for a brief period of time. Each time this happens the group will move more rapidly through the ensuing stages or they may even jump directly back to interdependence without experiencing the intervening stages.

The time it takes for any given group to progress through the stages varies greatly. Some groups will go through the process very rapidly in the first session, others less rapidly over a couple of sessions, and still other groups may evolve gradually over several sessions. The process depends on many variables such as (a) leadership style and skill, (b) the characteristics of the members, including personality and ability, (c) environmental circumstances, (d) the purpose of the group, and (e) the length of the group. Now let us examine these variables more closely.

VARIABLES AFFECTING GROUP DEVELOPMENT

Leadership Style and Skill

It is obvious that a leader's style and skill will affect the development of any group. An authoritarian leader who likes to make all the decisions as to what the group is to do and when, and who likes to keep close control of the group, will find that the group will remain in the dependent stage. Since all groups start at this stage and members may have no other experience, they are apt to be compliant and continue to do what they are told without question. As will be noted later in the discussion of leadership styles, members under authoritarian leadership do not make decisions nor are they given any responsibility. For some members, such as those that are depressed, such a situation is quite acceptable. But it can be seen that such an environment is not conducive to individuals becoming motivated, energized, or taking responsibility for their lives and behaviors.

A democratic leader, on the other hand, wants the members to become actively involved and stresses the attainment of an interdependent environment among group members and between group members and herself. In this role the leader tries to move out of the position of control and willingly accepts members' behaviors that are inherent in the stages of counterinterdependence, counterdependence, and independence in order for the group to evolve to a state of interdependence. This is done by being patient, accepting, responsive, tolerant, and good-natured, and by being aware of one's feelings and dealing with them within oneself. For example, when the group is floundering and the leader experiences great frustration, she controls the urge to jump in and say "Do this," or "Do it that way." Rather she lets the group struggle until they figure it out "their way." This is not to say that the leader cannot offer information or encouragement or be supportive in her efforts, but only to say that she will not do it for them. To do this requires many of the skills discussed under leader-therapist skills.

Characteristics of the Members

Often the progression of a group through its stages of development depends mainly on the functional level of the members. If a group is made up primarily of depressed individuals it will be extremely difficult to facilitate movement past the dependent stage. Rarely will they have the energy to be actively hostile, as is characteristic of the counterdependence stage, so when offered choices their most predictable response will be complete withdrawal. This is a less obvious form of hostility but one that ensures their dependence. In such a situation, the leader is forced to again become motivator, activator, and decision maker.

Conversely, if the membership includes may overconfident, verbal members they may be more than willing to accept or even seize control of the group from the leader. However, they may then become bogged down with infighting and one-upmanship in attempts to secure a single leadership position. This can prevent the group from moving on to interdependence and more group-shared productivity.

As a leader it is important to be aware of the types of members and to adjust one's expectations and behavior accordingly. Also, a group does not have to be in the interdependent stage in order to be a useful group. To have very depressed members respond to directions and participate, even if minimally and in a dependent way, may be an enormous progression for them. Groups, with chronic, low functioning members, may remain at this basic level but can continue to be useful in the important and therapeutic role of maintenance. Usually leader-therapists find they have a mix of functional levels among members which in and of itself can monitor and have facilitative effects.

Environment

As will be discussed later in the book, the environment plays a crucial role in the progress of any group. Many occupational therapy groups occur in hospitals where the medical model prevails. This model embodies the idea of being "done to." Patients are given medicines, food, housing, and rules, and in general are "looked after." They have little say in any of these aspects of their stay, so it is not surprising that when they come to an occupational therapy group they resist (counterindependence) having to take responsibility to make decisions. Many want to be "cured" and they expect the leader-therapist to do this, just as they have invested the physician with the ability and the responsibility to do this. In such an environment it takes skill and perseverance to work at inducing responsibility and engaging independent behaviors.

Purpose of the Group

The purpose or goals of a life skills group, for example, will differ in character from those of a classical psychotherapy group. In the life skills group, since the purpose will be to help the members learn or relearn some discreet behaviors, the leader is more likely to maintain a teacher-leader role. Because the leader has information to be imparted to the members, be it scenarios to be role-played or instructions on specific activities or techniques, this inequality of functions (teacher-learner) will keep the members in somewhat dependent roles vis-à-vis the leader for a longer period of time. In the psychotherapy group, where the goals are more vague and abstract, the leader may be completely nondirective right from the beginning, which can create high levels of anxiety in the members putting them immediately into the counterindependence stage. A third example, that of a decision making or consensus group, may help to clarify the point. The leader may give the group a list of variables to be rank-ordered according to certain principles. The group may quickly embrace the task and begin making decisions by majority vote. The leader may try to intervene to get the group to make decisions through discussion, but the suggestion is rejected because the group has very quickly moved to the counterdependence stage and although they may be vying for leadership among themselves, they are united in wanting to do it their way.

It can be seen from these examples how the goals and tasks of a group can affect the development of the group. It must be remembered though that each group goes through all the stages but the rate of passage varies widely with different groups and even within each session of the same group.

PHASES OF DEVELOPMENT

Through a review of the literature addressing the developmental sequence in small groups, Tuckman (1965) organized a model conceptualizing the behavioral changes occurring in all small groups throughout the life of the groups. His model includes four phases, *inclusion, control, affection, and functional,* also referred to as "forming," "storming," "norming," and "performing." In a later work, Tuckman and Jensen (1977) suggest that a fifth phase, *adjournment,* be added to the model. This stage of a group, also called the termination stage by others (Braaten, 1974/1975; Mann, 1967), is addressed in Chapter 7. By observing the developmental process of a group in more specific segments, Beck (1981) outlines nine themes with corresponding phases of group development. They are included here for both interest and comparison.

1. Creating a contract to become a group
2. Forging a group identity, resolving competitive work styles
3. Disclosure of individual identity, defining individual goals to be pursued in the group, establishing a cooperative and effective work style
4. Exploration of intimacy and closeness
5. Establishment of mutuality and equality
6. Autonomy of members from the formal leader
7. Self-confrontation in the context of interdependence, dissipation of roles
8. Assessment of learning, transfer of learning
9. Coping with separation and termination

The four phases of Tuckman's initial model have been selected for presentation here as they are more general and more closely parallel the stages of the authority cycle previously presented. The only difference between these two models is that Tuckman's fourth phase, the functional phase, encompasses the last two stages of the authority cycle, the independence and interdependence stages. Tuckman recognizes the differences among therapy groups, training groups, and natural groups by discussing separately the developmental phases in each. Since occupational therapists usually run groups considered to be combinations of the previously mentioned types, Tuckman's phases have here been combined to reflect this difference and will be discussed along three parameters, those of group structure, task behaviors, and therapy. A précis of the phases is offered in Table 2-1.

The four group phases will be examined through the hypothetical observations of a group with a specific task. This hypothetical group is meeting for the first time and, following opening remarks, has been asked to decide on a theme for a mural. Once this decision has been made, the members must produce a mural representative of the theme.

Inclusion Phase

Group Structure. According to Schultz (1986), the main concerns of members in the initial phase of any group are personally centered and have to

Table 2-1. CHARACTERISTICS OF
DEVELOPMENT SEQUENCE OF TASK GROUPS

Phase	Structure	Task	Therapy
Inclusion	Concern over belonging; overtalkative or withdrawn; self-centered; unawareness of and insensitivity to others; attention-getting behaviors	Check for ground rules; discover nature of task: what is expected, what is meaning of task, how task can be accomplished	Griping about institution; suspicious of whole situation; efforts to establish relationship with group leader
Control	Uneven interaction; lack of unity; intragroup conflict; acting-out behavior	Emotional response to task; challenge validity of task	Defensive behavior; ambivalent toward therapist; attempts to psychologically withdraw
Affection	Group unity and cohesion; mutual support, even interaction; assumes a family-life structure	Consensual group action; cooperation; acceptance of a common goal	Discussing personal problems; willingness to share, reveal, and probe; exploring dynamics of group
Functional	Functional role relatedness; group becomes a problem solving instrument; free and friendly	Constructive attempts at task completion; mutual task interaction; solutions emerge	Achieving understanding; gaining insights; modification and change in behaviors

Source: Adapted from B. W. Tuckman (1965), Developmental sequence in small groups. *Psychological Bulletin, 63,* 384–399.

do with the issue of belonging. Members' feelings reflect such concerns as, "Will I be accepted?" . . . "Will the others like me?" . . . "Do I know as much as the others?" . . . "If I speak will anyone listen?" . . . "Will I be different?" . . . "Will anyone like my suggestions for a theme?" . . . "What will the leader think of me?" Members deal with these anxious feelings by testing or trying out different behaviors in order to size up the situation. Herbert and Trist (1953) describe this initial stage as one of discovery. Seashore (1974) sees this stage as one where members form "collusive relationships" in an effort to establish some form of security. Members may be overtalkative or withdrawn, display a self-centered unawareness and insensitivity to others, try to impress the group by talking about outside experiences, display attention-getting behaviors, and pressure others into taking responsibility. These exploratory behaviors are all occurring in the context of trying to address the assigned task.

Task Behaviors. Initially, group members avoid taking responsibility for any decision making concerning the task. Member input abounds with such comments or questions as "I don't know," "What do the rest of you think?," "What do you mean by a theme?," "How big is the mural to be?," "How long do we have to do it?" These last three questions are likely to be addressed to the leader-therapist (dependence). Someone might then suggest, "Well, let's go around the table and everyone can give a suggestion." The next suggestion or question might follow as, "Shall we vote on the different ideas?"

Through all this the group is trying to discover how they are going to approach the task, what they need to know, and how the decision regarding a theme is to be made. Frequently questions will be directed to the leader-therapist, for guidance and as a means of checking out the ground rules.

Therapy. Tuckman (1965) reports behaviors characterizing this stage as being, in part, (a) griping about the institutional environment, (b) discussing peripheral problems, (c) discussing symptoms, (d) searching for the meaning of therapy, (e) attempting to establish rapport with the therapist, (f) intellectualizing, and (g) being suspicious and fearful of the new situation. In essence, the members of a therapy group at this stage are attempting to determine what will be expected of them, what they can expect to gain, whom can they relate to, and who is going to help them. For these reasons clients need plenty of time to go through these initial explorations and it is a mistake to hurry them or force them into close contact with others before they are ready (Battegay, 1986).

Control Phase

Group Structure. The outstanding characteristics of this stage are conflict, lack of unity, and testing-out behaviors. If the leader-therapist abdicates the leadership role in favor of the group assuming responsibility, then hostile feelings will develop between members and the leader. Members feel lost and uncertain ("Are we doing this the right way?" . . . "What is the right way?" . . . "Who is going to make the decisions?". . . "Who is going to tell us what to do?"). In order to deal with such anxieties some members will try to make the decisions ("I think we should do . . ." "What we should do now is . . ." "Let's just pick a topic and get started"). At this point the interaction in the group may become uneven (Bradford, 1964a) as some members withdraw (especially if they have made a suggestion and no one picked up on it); other members may disagree with such suggestions as are put forth and offer or not offer their own, while still others will compete for the leadership position abandoned by the leader-therapist. One observes competition rather than cooperation. Each member is trying to express his own individuality but often shying away from final decisions or from accepting responsibility for the group's actions. For instance, even the member trying for the leadership role may back off at the point where a member tries to give him the responsibility for the group. The comment, "I think we should take Joe's suggestion of spring for our theme," may elicit a response from Joe that goes, "Well, wait a minute, somebody might have a better idea."

Task Behaviors. Members display an emotional response to the task. They resist the task as a technique of therapy since it is unknown what will happen and how much of themselves they will be expected to disclose. The reaction to the task is frequently negative ("Who wants to do a mural anyway?" . . . "This is kid's stuff" . . . "I can't draw" . . . "We did this in kindergarten" . . . "This is dumb"). Such comments are most likely to be made at times of obvious conflict among members. It is a way of escaping the discomfort of the situation by evading the whole issue of task and decision making. The overall underlying reasoning is one of, "If we get rid of the task then we can also get rid of the conflict." Bion (1961) describes this period in a group as one of fight-flight. Most often he used the term to describe the interactions between the group and the leader, where members entered into conflict with the leader or they tried to withdraw psychologically from the whole situation. However, the term can also be applied to interactions among the group members when conflict or discord are present.

Therapy. The behaviors just described that are displayed by the members as they confront the task will obviously affect the therapeutic aspects of the group at this stage. Members tend to become argumentative, anxious, ambivalent toward the leader-therapist, and negative toward the group (Tuckman, 1965). Some acting out may occur as members are not sure of one another and are wary of the leader. Because of their fears and anxieties, members (at this point) are more concerned with what seems to them to be self-preservation than they are with treatment.

Fortunately for all involved, group development is such that invariably members not only survive the struggles of this phase, but gradually the very process they are involved in moves the group on to the next phase.

Affection Phase

Group Structure. This phase is characterized by positive feelings toward one another and the development of group unity and cohesion. Members really listen to what others are saying and consensual validation can be obtained. Members accept one another and their common purpose. However, there can be some negative feelings toward a member (or members) who is not responsive to the positive overtures being expressed. With harmony being of the utmost importance in this phase, members have low tolerance for those who do not support this norm. Cooperation, emotional support, cohesiveness, and permissiveness replace the competition displayed at the control phase (Bradford, 1964b). Members generally feel good about themselves and about the group. Positive feelings and comments are prevalent ("I like your idea" . . . "You are good at . . ." "I am . . . " "How shall we do . . . ?" "How do you feel about . . . ?" "Let's . . . ").

Trust is high, leading to genuine openness and sharing. As some members begin to disclose and confide personal information, others feel more comfortable in revealing themselves. Questioning and probing becomes an accepted norm. Members feel safe.

Task Behaviors. The control phase is usually followed by "consensual group action, cooperation, and mutual support" (Tuckman, 1965, p. 389). Let us say the hypothetical group survived the struggles of the control phase by agreeing on "Anger" as the theme for the group's mural and now they are ready to go on. In order to have some plan for their mural the members may talk about how they will actually do it as well as have a discussion about anger in general. This may point out how differently various members experience or react to anger. It is anticipated that they will support and encourage one another to make sure each member's contribution to the discussion or individual opinions and feelings about anger are heard and accepted. Interaction is fairly even with the more quiet members being encouraged to join in. Members have accepted the group and work to maintain a state of cohesion.

Therapy. During this phase members are motivated to share with one another and the tone of their interactions becomes more intimate, confidential, and revealing. The group takes on a "we-consciousness" with members showing concern and caring for one another. The willingness on the part of the members to reveal, probe, and respond allows the group to enjoy a period characterized by mutual exploration, sharing, and integration.

Functional Phase

Group Structure. By the time it reaches this phase the group has developed to a point where trust is high and members feel free to get on with the task in a unified group manner (Schroder & Harvey, 1963) without the emotional interference of anxieties. Members feel comfortable and able to use problem solving techniques to complete the task. Various members may assume directive roles at different times and these leadership functions are welcomed although not necessarily always acted on. The atmosphere in the group is a productive one, one of give-and-take.

Task Behaviors. Through the problem solving techniques that have emerged and using the information shared and evaluated in the previous phases, solutions emerge as to how the task will be accomplished. These solutions come from the process of asking for and giving suggestions (Bales, 1970) ("Who is good at drawing trees?". . . "If we keep the crayons in the middle then everyone can reach them" . . . "Some of us could work from the other side"). At this stage the group can become very caught up in the task and seem to have a vested interest in its completion. The members are now working collaboratively as a unit in an interdependent manner toward achieving the task and this goal becomes their main focus.

Therapy. This final stage of the group is characterized by a therapeutic atmosphere (Tuckman, 1965) and becomes a "work group" (Bion, 1961) where members achieve understanding, insight, and an analysis of some of their problems. In occupational therapy groups this last stage also often constitutes a discussion of how the task evolved, feedback to one another, how different members felt and what roles they played during the task, and what members learned about themselves and how they might do things differently. In task-therapy groups the format used in the group will depend on the type of task that is introduced. One format is for the members to work on a shared activity by themselves without any input or intervention by the leader-therapist. She will usually remain in the group or sit close by in order to observe the process and to intervene should it be necessary. Then when the group indicates that they have finished or if their time is up, the leader-therapist initiates a discussion. The discussion, as mentioned earlier, should involve an evaluation of how the group functioned during the activity. Depending on the nature of the activity the discussion may touch on issues such as: division of tasks and responsibilities, how members felt at different points during the activity, how members reacted to and interacted with one another, and what could have been done differently.

Another format is for the leader-therapist to take an active role in the group throughout. In this case the leader-therapist comments on the process and makes interventions as the group progresses. She makes observations, points out behaviors, encourages members to participate, share their feelings, and give feedback, and generally tries to get the members to examine the when, what, where, and how of the happenings during the session. A third format is for each member to do the task individually, such as a drawing or collage, and then when finished to share what they have done with the rest of the group. In this case it is best if the leader-therapist does the activity along with the members. This gives her the opportunity to be aware of what the members are experiencing, to be a role model for performing the task, downplay her leadership role, and be able to observe what is going on in the group without appearing to be sitting and watching.

Not every group will move through the stages as clearly or as smoothly as has been presented here. However, groups do develop in the order of these stages, but as with human development each group will do so at its own speed. As noted in the discussion of the authority cycle, groups can also get bogged down at any one stage or revert back to an earlier stage. For example, even as our hypothetical group reaches the functional phase and begins to work on the task, members may experience feelings of anxiety similar to those experienced during the inclusion phase because they feel the immediacy of the expectations to actually work and produce. This makes sense in that it is quite like a new group. Up until this point the group has been involved in teaching, sharing, and problem solving. Now the members are expected to "do something" and many of the concerns noted during the inclusion phase are triggered all over again. However, the established norm of acceptance and the mood of cohesiveness and unity enjoyed by the group at this stage serve as strong supports in enabling members to feel safe in taking this next stop of "doing." It should be noted that the task of the group is not usually an issue in group development. Our hypothetical group could have been involved in other kinds of tasks and the group development would basically follow the same pattern. Only the rate of development and the time spent in the various stages would differ.

SUMMARY

A small group meets the requirements of a system by having members as the "parts," the personalities of the members as the "properties," and the feelings and interactions among the members as the "relationships." In addition, a group is believed to be an open system since it does not maintain a constant state of homeostasis but is constantly developing and changing. In considering the four types of systems — natural, designed physical, designed abstract, and human activity — small groups fall into the last category.

Any ongoing group is in a constant process of development. The rate and nature of this development depends on several variables such as the skill and style of leadership, the characteristics of the members, the environment, the purpose of the group, the length of the group, the interactions among the members, and the interactions between the leader and the members. These variables will be of more or less importance in the development of different groups.

Group development can be seen to encompass distinct stages. The model presented here includes four phases, these being inclusion, control, affection, and functional. At each of these phases it is informative and useful to direct your observations along three parameters. By focusing on these three parameters (group structure, task behaviors, and therapy) an observer is more likely to be aware of all aspects of the group's development. Although all groups grapple with the four stages each group will do so in different ways and within a different time frame.

CHAPTER 3

Group Dimensions

All groups require warmth and protection — some more than others.
— ALFRED BENJAMIN

Quite different from the structured and formalized phase development approach to group development is Dimock's (1985a) framework of group dimensions. He emphasizes the importance of understanding the factors that affect the development or growth of a group as a means of guiding one's observations of process. Dimock states that "by observing, understanding and giving attention to these areas groups can improve their procedures, accomplish higher level tasks, and enable members to satisfy more of their developmental needs" (Dimock, 1985a, p. 1). For Dimock this framework takes the form of five dimensions: climate, interaction, involvement, cohesion, and productivity. All five areas are discussed. The climate or environment of a group is a first consideration and because it is the one component which can be directly affected by the attentiveness of the leader-therapist, this component will be given special emphasis.

CLIMATE

Most people concern themselves with the state of the living room, family room, or recreation room whenever they are going to have friends over. It is usual to want the room to appear inviting, look tidy and attractive and, hopefully, be comfortable. For the same reasons, group leaders should be equally concerned with the group room before members arrive. Barris (1982) concludes that the environment can play a role in affecting a person in three areas: developing interests and values, communicating performance expectations, and affecting participation in future environments. The surroundings in which a group is held can exert the same effects as well as having a strong influence on the group process (Levine, 1979; Palazzolo, 1981; Shaw, 1976). Unfortunately, this is an aspect that is often ignored or overlooked by leader-therapists. Some leader-therapists are not aware of the importance of the environment to the overall functioning of the group. Others were aware at one time but through habit, work constraints, familiarity, or carelessness, they have ceased to see this as an area of focus or concern. Still others have a sense that "things have always worked this way so why change?" The leader-therapist needs to be sensitive at all times to dynamics in the group that may be a result of environmental factors. Such factors can have an effect at any time during the group and so the leader-therapist must keep this possibility in mind throughout the group, and not only at the beginning.

ENVIRONMENTAL FACTORS

There are two major environmental factors to be considered: (1) physical factors, and (2) emotional factors (Dimock, 1985a). Under physical factors the following will be discussed: (a) space, (b) temperature, (c) seating arrangements, (d) sound, and (e) dress. Emotional factors involve the mood of (a) the leader, (b) the group, and (c) individual members.

Physical Factors

Space. The amount of space available and how it is utilized is of utmost importance in setting up your group. Levine (1979) suggests "the room where the group meets and its set-up can greatly enhance or distract from the group's development" (p. 7). Ideally, you will be in a position to select and furnish the room in which you will hold your group. Realistically, you will probably be allotted the room or the space. Most likely, as an occupational therapist, you will hold your group in a room that is used by different therapists at various times for other activities such as assessments, treatment, other groups, and social events.

Given the ideal situation, what kind of selections would you make? Some group leaders feel that if you have windows in your room you will have noise and distractions. This may be true for certain situations, but it is the writer's belief that the light and feeling of openness more than compensates for these drawbacks. If you have a bright, windowed room, you are more likely to induce a "bright" group. A windowless room tends to give a dingy, closed-in feeling, which in turn is apt to encourage only a "closed" unproductive group.

Space is an important factor to consider in setting up your group (Palazzolo, 1981). You will need enough space so that you can organize your group comfortably either around a table or seated in a circle without a table. A sectioned table is sometimes useful so that when it is not needed it can be easily set aside in the unused corners of the room rather than take up most of one end or side of the room. You will also need enough space so that group members can space themselves comfortably apart from one another and not feel that their personal space is invaded. However, you do want members seated close enough together so that interaction is encouraged. Hall (1966) sets intimate distance as being 6 to 8 inches and personal distance as being 1½ to 4 feet. You need also to keep in mind that you may want to easily maneuver extra chairs in and out of the group, say, for role playing.

Like Goldilocks, for the *ideal* situation, you want a room that is not too big and not too small. Too large a room can detract from feelings of closeness and cohesion and too small a room can cause members to feel hemmed in or trapped (Bertcher & Maple, 1977). Often, therapists solve the problem of a large space by organizing one corner of the room into the group area. In doing so the therapist provides walls and hence "protection" on at least two sides of the group and thus a little more sense of security for the members.

The space problems can also be related to scheduling and the needs of other staff members. The situation can arise where the room in which you routinely hold your sessions has been appropriated by another staff member for a special presentation. On discovering this conflict in scheduling it may be suggested that you could hold your group in the "small room across from the office." The problem this presents is one of territoriality (Wolfe & Proshansky, 1974), not in the sense of your "territory" as a professional (although this could be an issue) but in the sense of the group members' territory. When hospitalized, clients give up the familiar territory of their homes and all their personal places such as "my room," "my place at the table," "my closet" and so on. In hospital they establish new territories, spaces, and places which they can feel are theirs. The "group room" can having meaning in this context as a place they are familiar with and feel comfortable in. Addressing this point Battegay (1986) says "the room does not merely belong to the group; it is a part of it" (p. 143). He goes on to emphasize the importance of establishing a group room that remains constant. So before accepting the quick solution of the room across from the office, it would be in the best interests of the group to pursue the issue for alternatives offering a better choice.

- *Alternative 1.* Try to get the group that is having the presentation in the group room to relocate. It is possible that the persons responsible for arranging the presentation were not aware that your group was scheduled to be held in the same room at the same time. Bringing this to their attention as well as the fact that a presentation can be successful in a variety of settings (e.g., classrooms or conference rooms) may be all that is needed to effect the change. A little assertiveness may be appropriate!

- *Alternative 2.* Try to find a room that is similar to the regular group room. Perhaps the room across from the office is not the only room to consider. Check with other members of the staff for suggestions. They may be aware of a schedule change that frees up a more suitable room.

- *Alternative 3.* Hold the group at a different time but in the usual room. Although it is definitely best to hold your group at the same time each session, it may be less disruptive to change the time than to change the room. This is especially true if the alternative room is extremely unsuitable. Before doing this, of course, it is essential to check if the new time conflicts with other events scheduled for the members or the leader-therapist.

- *Alternative 4.* If the above choices are not possible, then you may decide to go ahead and hold the group in the small room available across from the office. Having made this decision try to make the room as conducive to the group's needs as possible and be prepared for the members to be somewhat distracted by the new surroundings. It is likely to take members longer to feel both comfortable and a part of the group. Sharing your own frustrations about the situation with the members will demonstrate your concern and can induce more cooperative and accepting attitudes all around.

- *Alternative 5.* You may decide that the available room is really too small and since you cannot find any other space your only alternative is to cancel the session for the day. Should you decide to do this, be sure that you or a reliable staff member contact each member to inform them of the circumstances and the reasons for the cancellation. Some members will be disappointed and others may feel relieved. Either way they need a full explanation, preferably from the group leader or another staff member. If it can be avoided, do not ask a group member to tell the other members, as this can raise all sorts of brooding questions in the minds of the members. They may also feel that the group cannot be very important if you do not take the time to inform them of the change yourself.

Temperature. It goes without saying that the room needs to be well-ventilated with a comfortable temperature. The latter may be quite difficult to achieve for all of your members. Some members may prefer a cooler room than others due to their medication or their natural preference. It is quite usual for older clients to prefer a warm room temperature. It is a good idea to check this out with your members and not rely totally on your own comfort level or preference. A room that is very warm is likely to cause clients to feel groggy and not too energetic or motivated.

The chances are that if you are working in an institution you will have very little control over the temperature in the room. So what should you do? Sometimes you will have access to a window that opens and this can help to relieve the stuffiness or cut down on the temperature if it is felt by the group members that the room is too hot. It if does not prove to be too distracting, then opening the door may allow some exchange of air. In doing this, you may have to decide which is the most disruptive of the two situations — to be too hot or to be distracted by what is going on outside the door.

If you are conducting a group session that will require physical movement, such as an exercise group or even an active warm-up exercise, it is important to be aware of the temperature factor and try to adjust it to the needs of the group. Opening a window or the door while engaged in these sorts of activities usually does not cause any disruption to the group.

Seating Arrangements. How and where clients sit in a group may appear to be very mundane issues. In actual fact, they are issues of consequence and can greatly affect the dynamics in the group (Wolfe & Proshansky, 1974). The type of seats, how they are arranged, and where clients choose to sit are all significant issues and require the attention of the group leader. Research by Pellegrini (1971) demonstrated that sitting at the head of a rectangular table can have a significant effect on all the other persons seated at the table. He found that the person who occupies the end position was rated higher on dimensions such as talkativeness, dominance, persuasiveness, self-confidence, leadership, and intelligence. Looking at Figure 3-1 one can see how all the group members are focused on the man seated at the end of the table. It is also interesting to note how the members seated distant from the focal person tend to lean forward in attempts to be included. As leader-therapist of a small group where you wish to encourage participation and downplay your authority role, it is particularly important to avoid sitting in this head position yourself. Unfortunately, members will invariably avoid this seat too, leaving it for the leader. In this case it is best to ask a member to switch places with you before starting the group.

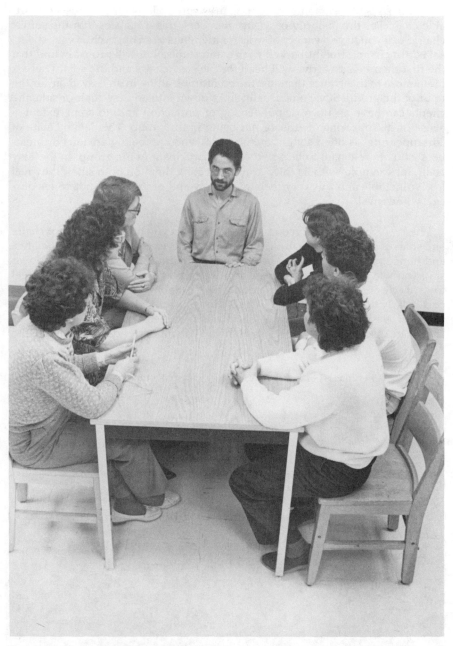

Figure 3-1. Focus of members when one of the group sits in the head position.

Type of seats. Most members coming into a group look for the most comfortable chair. For the majority of group members, this translates into the softest chair! So, if you have a variety of seats for members to sit on, such as easy chairs, sofas, armchairs, straight-backed chairs, and stools, you will probably find that the first members to arrive will head for the easy chairs and the sofa. There is often more to this choice than just the comfort of sitting in an easy chair for the hour of the group. Since one usually sinks down into an easy chair or sofa, the clients can have an unconscious feeling of protection and, to some extent, a sense of disappearing, that is, of not being in the group. This feeling state of "disappearing" is often sought by members who are feeling anxious or members who are reluctant to be a part of or a participant in the group. In the easy chair, for example, with its thick arms protecting them on both sides, they feel less vulnerable and this very feeling of safety and protection tends to encourage withdrawal.

Levels. As can be observed in Figure 3-2, when you have a mixture of chairs and sofas of different types the actual seating surfaces will be of varying heights, and hence your members will be sitting at different levels. This up-and-down situation will affect the interactions in the group as well as how members feel toward one another. Take the situation where a member is feeling depressed or particularly down and is seated in a soft, low-cushioned easy chair or even on the floor, beside a member on a solid straight-backed and thus a higher-level chair. The discrepancy in the levels of the two members tends to accentuate the

Figure 3-2. "Unevenness" of members caused by different sitting heights.

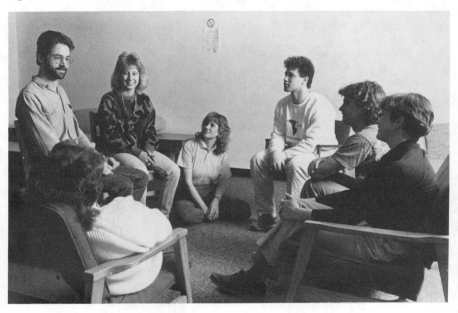

situation and cause the lower-level member to feel even more depressed or down. The best one can do is to have all the chairs in the group be of similar, if not the same type. This removes competition for the soft seats, any distractions caused by "who is sitting in which chair," and problems related to differences in eye levels.

An example of the fact that seating can be an issue was emphasized in a group led by the author and a cotherapist. Since the experience was to be a weekend group, the plan was to sit on pillows on the floor in the hopes of being more comfortable. Twelve large pillows covered in material of a blue and black design were available and just the right number for the expected 12 group members. The coleaders, realizing the need for two more pillows, picked up two available sleeping pillows, took them along to sit on, and began the group. Being bed pillows both had ordinary white pillowcases. The group was slower in getting started than had been expected with members seeming a little tense and tentative. After about an hour, a member finally asked what was the meaning behind the white pillows that the leaders were sitting on. As soon as the question was asked the group came alive with many other members joining in the querying. It was obvious that most group members had been concerned and preoccupied with the pillows from the beginning of the group. Once it was explained that the white pillows held no significance the feeling tone of the group became more relaxed and comfortable. Sitting on pillows on the floor, as shown in Figure 3-3, can lessen the formality of a group and promote intimacy. However, it is not really recommended for a therapeutic group as not every one

Figure 3-3. An informal atmosphere.

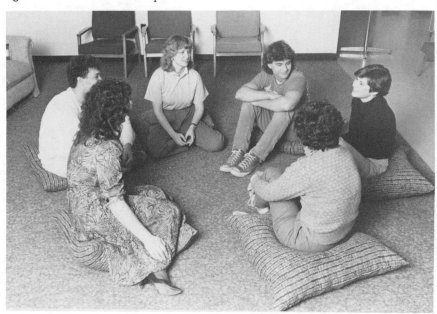

feels comfortable sitting on the floor for an hour and you do risk members sprawling, lying down, or falling asleep.

Configuration. Make every effort to have your group members seated in a circle (Figure 3-4), as this encourages and facilitates communication among the members. Heap (1977) notes that "interaction is most likely to occur where participants are able to see each other" (p.122). Verbal groups are most always seated in a circle without a table and if there is a table it is frequently a low coffee table. However, task groups, where members are involved in doing an activity, tend to be conducted with members seated around a table, as in Figure 3-5. In this situation the table is mainly utilitarian in supplying a surface for members to work on while carrying out the requirements of the task.

In discussing the pros and cons of using tables in groups, Levine (1979) notes that a table can have several other useful purposes. It offers support to group

Figure 3-4. The most facilitative seating arrangement for group members.

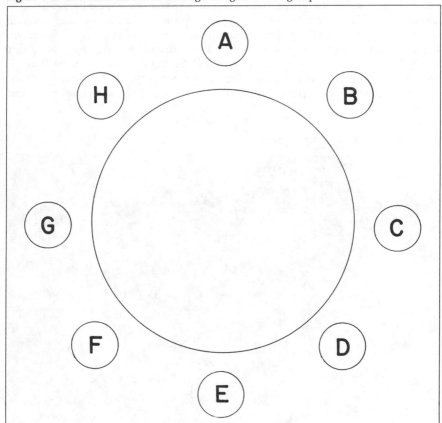

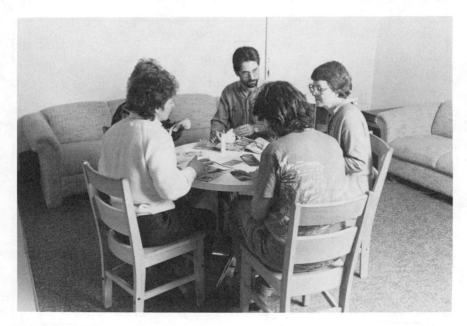

Figure 3-5. Making a collage.

members, it gives them something to lean on, a place to put their hands, as well as serving as a link between the group members. In groups with children or adolescents a table can often serve as a divider to keep antagonistic members separated and thereby reduce opportunities for physical contact. Finally, members who are feeling shy, self-conscious, or nervous may find the table to be partial protection from physically exposing themselves to others.

If it is decided that a table should be used, then the importance of finding a round table must be emphasized even though it seems that the tables available in most facilities tend to be rectangular. There are drawbacks to having round tables, and more practical staff members will be quick to point them out. For example, round tables do not fit into square rooms very easily. They cannot be compactly pushed to the side or into the corner. Round tables cannot be enlarged by connecting two of them the way that square or rectangular ones can. Also, with the round table usually being all one piece, with a small group the table may be considered to be too large.

If one looks at Figure 3-6 one can see how the seating configuration can affect the type of interactions that occur. With this rectangular positioning and eight members, one can see that two subgroups, A-B-C and F-G-H, may be formed. This possibility exists because members will most often talk to (a) someone they can easily make eye contact with, or (b) someone who is sitting close to them. It is Sommer's (1962) finding that people prefer to engage in conversation with persons sitting across from them than with persons sitting beside

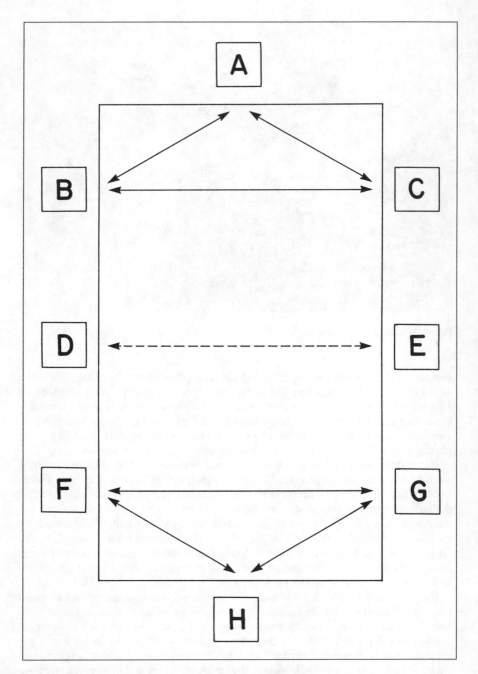

Figure 3-6. Effect of seating configuration on communication patterns.

them. The above two tenets hold true for the three members of each of these two groups. This does not mean that the two groups will be active at the same time during the session, but when members in these locations do interact it is likely to be in the directions indicated. It may be argued that G is also close to E or that D is close to B. This is true, of course, but the second tenet does not hold true for these pairs in that they cannot easily make eye contact. In Figure 3-7 the two members centered on the sofas appear left out of the conversation and are too distant from each other to interact comfortably. To make eye contact is really what we mean when we say "I can see you," and if we say "I can't see you," we usually mean, "I can't see your eyes."

For G or B to make the half-turn to speak to the member beside them requires a greater risk than to merely glance slightly to the left or right in hopes of catching another member's eyes and thus finding someone to speak to. Of course, it can be seen that it would not be possible for G to make eye contact with C unless E moves back out of the line of vision or G moves forward. What usually happens is that two members of a group who are seated in positions such as G and C rarely interact with each other.

It is true that some people have difficulty making or maintaining eye contact, but even persons who do find it difficult to make eye contact like to know that the other person involved is facing them so that if they do glance up they feel some contact.

There is more opportunity and it is much easier for members to make eye contact when seated in a circle. It can be seen in Figure 3-8 that the angles be-

Figure 3-7. Interaction problems with poor seating arrangements.

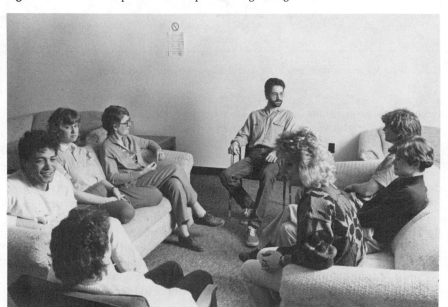

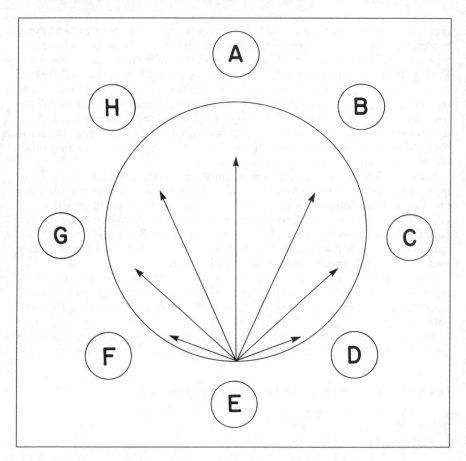

Figure 3-8. A circle contributes to equalization of interactive possibilities.

tween each group member from, for example, the position of E, are almost equal. These angles would be the same for the other members as well in relation to the rest of the group.

Sound. Often a group leader is at the mercy of the physical layout of the department in terms of finding a suitable room in which to hold the group. Rarely does a department enjoy the luxury of having a special group room. Surrounding sounds that may not disrupt the other activities that a room is used for are often very distracting if one is conducting a group. Sometimes a group room is formed by dividing a large room with a divider of some sort such as a folding wall. Although such dividers may remove visual distractions, they do not keep out such sounds as music, voices, or laughter. Such noises can be very distracting as well as making it difficult for members to hear one another. Also, if a group member is sharing something very important or painful to himself, it can be very upsetting if this type of disclosure coincides with a burst of laughter or a blare of music from the adjoining area. Such an occurrence can often set off a burst of laughter in the group, especially from members who are feeling tense and anxious. Such outbursts can be quite inappropriate in relation to the process going on in the group at the time. So, as much as possible, try to control the exterior environment so that it, as well as the environment in the room, is conducive to feelings of safety among members.

Dress. Dressing for a group does not really differ from the general requirements of dressing in good taste for the other aspects of a therapist's work. Just as clients give messages to others by the way that they dress, so do we as leader-therapists give messages to them. Clothing can indicate attitudes, moods, personality characteristics, self-esteem, and emotional states. The way that we dress can also affect our interactions with and influence on others. Brilhart (1974) warns, "For better or worse, we ignore the impact of our adornment in small groups at the peril of being less effective than desired" (p. 49).

Practically and socially one's dress should suit the activity of the session. If the group is going to be doing some exercises or is expected to work while sitting on the floor, then slacks are going to be more appropriate than a tight skirt. For a group outing to a restaurant or community event, appropriate attire for the time and place serves as a role model and reminder to clients to try and look their best since it is in their own best interest.

Whether you are male or female, as a leader-therapist you should avoid wearing clothing that has sexual connotations or promotes sensuality. Often clients are grappling with sexual problems or younger members are attempting to cope with identity issues. Provocative clothing in and of itself can be disturbing and the cause of increased anxiety.

Emotional Factors

General Mood. The emotional climate of your group is going to fluctuate from session to session. One should never assume that, because members are cooperative and cheerful one day, they will arrive in the same state the next day. Pointing this out, Bradford (1978a) cautions, "In a sense, a group reforms each time it meets" (p. 4). Group members usually participate in a variety of treatment programs so they will be having other therapeutic experiences in addition to your group. Some of these experiences may be stressful and upsetting, some may be exhilarating and stimulating. When members come to group directly from these various experiences their moods will reflect a variety of feeling states as well. Because of this it may take some members longer to adjust and get into the group than it will others.

A group is basically a new entity at each session and therefore it is not possible to carry over the mood from one meeting to the next. It can even be difficult to pick up a discussion from where it left off at a previous session. It is a common occurrence for the most important issue of the session to be brought up just a few minutes before the group is scheduled to close. This can happen for a couple of reasons. The member may find it a difficult topic to discuss and so spends the group time getting up the courage to bring it up and, as time runs out, the pressure results in the member finally saying something. Or it could be that it is only by the end of the session that the member feels the emotional climate is such that he feels safe to share his issue. Such situations can present real dilemmas. Notwithstanding the problems with carry-over you might suggest that, since there is so little time left, the discussion be held over and brought up at the beginning of the next group. It is likely that in the interim the member will have an opportunity to discuss the issue elsewhere and so it will no longer be of the same relevance to him or the group. If it is still an issue for him, you may find that he is reluctant to pursue it in the following group as he does not sense the same emotional climate as he did previously. It is best not to pressure the member or belabor the point at such a time but rather to wait and see if he brings it up later when he feels more comfortable.

Your group will not always be in a good mood nor should they be. The purpose of most groups is to deal with problems and problem behaviors. For most people this is tough work and can be very painful. If the emotional climate is one of openness, caring, and sharing, then this will be felt as being supportive to members who may be struggling with themselves or with other stressful issues.

Mood of the Leader. It is important to realize that the leader-therapist, by virtue of her status, has the power to influence the emotional climate of the group. If you are enthusiastic, open, and caring, you have a better chance of eliciting these behaviors from your group members. If you are quiet, reserved, and cautious, it is most likely that group members will follow suit. New members especially look to you for clues and guidelines of what behaviors are acceptable and desired. Seldom will they ask but more often will be guided by the leader-therapist's behavior. Be aware of your own affect. Make sure that your facial expression is congruent with your behavior; otherwise you can give group members double messages. For example, if your face portrays annoyance but you behave in an accepting way, your group members will not know which of these messages to react to and so they may withdraw. Sometimes, we have facial expressions that we are not aware of. This writer once worked with a student who always looked rather angry — even when she was feeling happy. Her constant dour facial expression caused the patients to be very wary of her and hence they found her unapproachable. Once she was made aware of this incongruency, she worked hard at changing her facial expression, with some positive results.

Mood of the Group. It is important to have an unremitting awareness of and sensitivity to the mood of the group. There is little that is more frustrating to group members than when they are, on the whole, feeling down or upset to have the leader-therapist ignore their mood and proceed to be bright and enthusiastic. What is more likely to elevate the group's mood is for you to recognize and acknowledge the group's feelings by labeling what you sense, remark that "everyone seems a little down today," and encourage the members to discuss the situation. Sometimes, an incident has occurred on the ward or elsewhere in the treatment center that is of concern to the group members. Until the issue is dealt with, it is likely to be difficult and unproductive to proceed with the group task.

Mood of Individual Members. It is rare that you will find all group members in the same mood or frame of mind when they arrive for a group meeting. Since they will all have had different experiences prior to your group, perhaps some positive and some negative, it is important that you recognize these differences among the members. Some leader-therapists find it productive to actually check out with each member how they are feeling at the beginning of the group. Others may find it more meaningful to comment on the moods of individual members as they sense them. For example, on noticing that a member is particularly quiet, you might say something like, "Mary, you seem unusually quiet today, is something bothering you?," or "John, you look rather down, are you feeling sad?," or "It's nice to see you smiling, Ann, are you feeling happy?" If an individual member is in a pronounced mood of sadness or happiness, it can affect the other members. A very depressed member can bring other members down. Also, an exuberant member can be irritating to other members if they are trying to cope with some heavy feelings. Dealing with such situations will be addressed more thoroughly in Chapter 8.

INTERACTION

The frequency and types of communication among members in small groups are affected by many factors. One factor is the size of the group. The larger the group the more likelihood there is of having nonparticipating members (Schwartzberg, Howe, & McDermott, 1982). Often individuals, even those who could be described as confident, are reluctant to speak out in a group and they are even more reluctant to speak out if the group is large. On this point Heap (1977) concludes that as the size of the group increases, "Fewer and fewer members say more and more, while more and more members say less and less" (p. 135). It should always be remembered that members of a therapeutic group are usually feeling a certain degree of anxiety, which in and of itself can be inhibiting.

The number of staff that are present in a group can affect the types of interactions that occur. As the number of staff increases so do the member-to-staff and staff-to-member communications (Schwartzberg, Howe, & McDermott, 1982). So in order to encourage member-to-member interactions the ratio of staff to members should be considered and maintained at an appropriate level. The staff-to-member ratio can be a problem in clinical settings where teaching is a mandate and several students require group experience at the same time. This situation can be handled by having certain students observe the group through a one-way mirror, although this arrangement does not afford the students an opportunity to practice leadership skills. Another practice employed by some clinicians is to have the students sit in the room but outside the group. In the experience of the writer this latter method can be inhibiting and disruptive to the naturalness and effective functioning of the group.

A key factor that affects the frequency of interaction is the type of task in which the members are involved. Some tasks, by their nature, require greater interaction among members than do others. Through the process of activity analysis the leader-therapist should be able to decide, with some degree of certainty, that given this situation activity A will elicit more interaction than activity B. Try to keep this important factor in mind whenever you are selecting a task for any group. Task analysis will be further discussed in Chapter 13.

The development of active subgroups or dyads in a group can affect the level of participation by the remaining members in the group (Bales, Strodtbeck, Mills, & Roseborough, 1951). Members are hesitant to break in on a conversation that is going on between only two or three members of the group and this very avoidance tends to perpetuate interactions exclusively among the subgroup or dyad. An intervention by the leader-therapist is sometimes required to bring about a more generalized and more inclusive discussion.

The more group members interact among themselves the more likely is the group to grow and develop. It is also the case that the more members interact and get to know one another the more likely they are to like one another and so feel inclined to further interaction. As was discussed under Environmental Factors the way in which the physical setting is arranged can greatly affect the level and areas of interaction. When members are seated so that they can clearly see one another they are more likely to interact. It was also noted previously that the emotional climate is a major factor in enhancing or inhibiting the interaction level among members. Members who feel secure and accepted in the group are more likely to interact in a more meaningful way by expressing their thoughts and feelings or sharing their problems and concerns.

A critical factor, not to be overlooked, is that a great deal of the interaction occurring between and among members consists of nonverbal messages. Research by Mehrabian (1971) indicates that only 7 percent of communication is verbal, leaving 93 percent to occur through nonverbal channels. These nonverbal messages are not only a part of the interaction process but they also can greatly affect the process. A member's smile may be enough support to encourage another member to speak, or, conversely, an unfriendly glance may be sufficient to deter a member from participating. Nonverbal messages are constantly being given and received by all members in the group, as illustrated in Figure 3-9. All the output messages of each member are being received as input by all the other members and each member will be affected by these nonverbal messages in different or similar ways. For example, if member A raises his voice when speaking, this may intimidate some members who will respond by withdrawing, while other members may respond by becoming angry or argumentative. Member A may only be trying to make a benign point, but

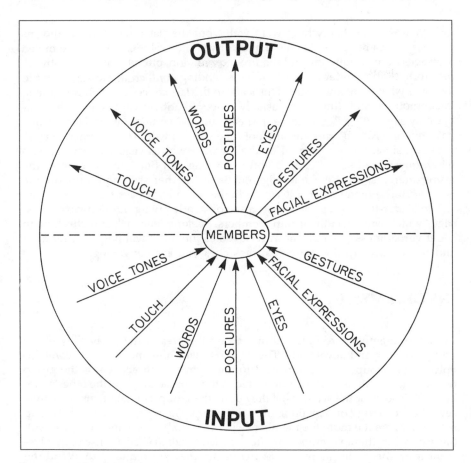

Figure 3-9. Flow of nonverbal messages.

because of his raised voice the point can be lost as others react only to the tone of his voice. If member B is restless and constantly fidgeting, the other group members may tend to avoid interacting with B, thinking he may be feeling upset and not wanting to risk upsetting him further. On the other hand, when a member speaks and notices looks of interest and nods of agreement from others, he is likely to be encouraged to continue speaking and interacting.

Brilhart (1974) presents three concepts that he believes to be especially relevant to small group interaction. First, it is not possible to *not* communicate. Each member, at all times, is giving out messages and cues nonverbally. The way one sits, looks, moves or does not move, gestures, and speaks all tell others a great deal about oneself. Second, the meaning perceived from the nonverbal message is always received as being more significant than the meaning conveyed by the words. A member attempting to deny a disastrous weekend pass may say, "It was great. Everything went well," but the flat tone of voice and his downcast eyes belie his statement and convey the real message. These mixed messages occur frequently and require intervention, often by the leader-therapist, to help the sender realize that he is sending conflicting messages and to discover what he really means. This leads to the last concept, which is that feelings, emotions, and attitudes are usually conveyed nonverbally. A difficult member may say that he is glad to be in the group and certainly intends to participate, but his crossed arms, defiant look, and clipped words tell another story. A common situation is presented by the member who is visibly upset but who when questioned says, "There's nothing wrong, I'm fine." In such a case the leader-therapist must make a judgment as to whether she should pursue the issue with the member or if it would be better to let it pass for the moment.

The leader-therapist is, of course, also constantly giving out nonverbal messages which will affect the group members. Seeking feedback and checking to see if verbal messages have been received as intended will help you monitor and be sensitive to the nonverbal messages you are conveying.

INVOLVEMENT

The more members are involved in a group the greater the probability of the group growing and developing. The degree to which members will become involved in a group is directly related to the degree of attractiveness the group holds for them. Members will be attracted to the group if they like the other members, the leader, or the activities; if they think the group can help them; or if they see others enjoying or benefiting from the group. The more attractive the group is for members the more the members will become absorbed and occupied with the group. In a therapy setting it is often more difficult to elicit a sense of involvement from the group members, as frequently they are required to attend the group as part of their treatment program. Because of this the members of a therapeutic group, at least initially, may be resistive and disinterested. It is therefore essential that you exert every effort to present the group and the idea of attending the group in a positive way. Needless to say, the group will have to live up to any such assertions for the members to remain involved. Therefore the tasks and activities selected should be creative, interesting, and engaging.

Most leader-therapists will be able to judge the degree of involvement of individual members by their attendance, their level of participation, and the degree of interest they show in the task or other members. If the members appear uninvolved or apathetic it is important to assess the situation carefully to determine why the group is unattractive to the members. Involvement may be low due to lack of interest in the task, lack of obvious relevance of the task, the low energy level of the members, the monopolizing of input by one or two members, or an incompatible mix of member interests and personalities. Including the members in the decision making processes in the group as much as possible is a way to engage members, increase their feelings of competency, and therefore encourage involvement.

COHESION

Dimock (1985a) believes that the degree of cohesiveness present in a group is directly related to and partly determined by the degree of involvement felt by the members. Members who together choose to be actively involved in a group will experience a sense of "we-ness" and solidarity that is known as cohesion. This unity results from members sharing themselves, trying to understand others, accepting others, and allowing interest and caring for others to develop. Nixon (1979) discusses at length the problems encountered in attempting to define the term *cohesiveness*. The difficulties arise, he says, due to the lack of agreement among small group investigators as to the conceptual and operational meaning of the term. For his purposes he sees cohesiveness as a "basic group property . . . reflecting overall member attraction to a group as a whole" (Nixon, 1979, p. 78). It is seen as the sum or the coming together of the feelings of attraction felt by all the group members for the group. It is a feeling state that can be sensed when members like being together and like what they are doing.

Cohesion can be a strong and productive force in influencing the behavior and attitudes of group members (Shaw, 1976). Members enjoy and feel comfortable in a cohesive environment and will behave in ways to maintain rather than disrupt such a state of togetherness. Rudestam (1982) says: "The more cohesive a group is, the more group control there is over the attitudes and actions of its members, the more conformity and commitment to group norms, and the greater acceptance of group values" (p. 19). A cohesive group has a climate of trust. This permits members to feel secure and be more open in sharing thoughts and feelings, including the giving and receiving of both positive and negative feedback. A trusting environment also fosters the expression of opposing views, ideas, and beliefs so that a more thorough examination of issues is possible.

A cohesive group is usually a productive and growing group but there are times when the feelings of we-ness become too strong (Fisher, 1974). This is evident when the members become closed to new members or new directions and invest their energies only in protecting the status quo. An intense feeling of unity can prevent members from disagreeing or behaving in any manner that could possibly produce conflict. Members become hesitant to give honest feedback if it is not positive. They may back away from personal problems or issues that they see as potential areas of discomfort for any member. Such an environment prevents further growth or development of the group as an entity and of the members individually.

PRODUCTIVITY

Productivity, although somewhat different from the other group dimensions, is none the less an important aspect of any group. Members need to feel that the time they spend in the group is worthwhile, that it is productive for the group and for themselves personally. This is best accomplished if the members understand the goals or purpose of the group, if they are able to integrate their own goals into the goals or purposes of the group, and if they see the group moving toward accomplishing these ends.

As mentioned in the section on stages of development, the functional phase is the fourth stage and that is why a mature group is generally more productive than a young group. A group may grapple with some or all of the other dimensions and phases before achieving the satisfaction of end productivity. The interdependent relationship between cohesiveness and productivity should be emphasized. It was noted above that a cohesive group is usually a productive group and the converse is also true: A productive group is usually a cohesive group (Fisher, 1974). These two components of a group affect each other reciprocally and an increase in one tends to produce an increase in the other.

In therapy groups, productivity cannot be defined as clearly or easily as it can be in a straight task group. A task may be used in a therapy group, but since it frequently serves as a catalyst, and is not an end in itself, it would be the results of this catalytic effect that would be seen as productive or unproductive. This is an important reason to select the task with care.

SUMMARY

The importance of the effects of the environment on the process and functioning of a group cannot be overemphasized. Many of the points made in this chapter may appear to be based in common sense but it is surprising how many of them, through habituation or nonthinking, can be ignored. Leader-therapists must remember that they themselves have participated in and are familiar with the process of therapeutic groups, but for many of their members it will be a first-time experience. What leader-therapists know, understand, and expect is likely to be all new for the members. To allay some of the anxieties and fears of the clients the leader-therapist should try to make the setting as comfortable, inviting, and conducive to well-being as possible.

There are five main factors that can affect the growth or development of a group: climate, interaction, involvement, cohesion, and productivity. The climatic factor encompasses both the physical and emotional aspects of the environment. Physical factors that the leader-therapist should pay close attention to when planning or organizing a group are space, temperature, seating, configuration, sound, and dress.

It is the responsibility of the leader-therapist to make sure that the room is of appropriate size, that the seats are comfortable and arranged to encourage easy interaction, that the room is neither too hot nor too cold, and that outside noise or disruption is avoided. Emotionally, the leader-therapist must be aware of her own mood during any given group just as she must be sensitive to the mood of the group as a whole and to each member individually. This awareness of mood is crucial to understanding the process that unfolds in each group.

Since a purpose of every group is to have members relate to one another, it is important to know what promotes and, conversely, what inhibits interaction. It is the role of the leader-therapist to monitor all interactions, both verbal and nonverbal, to insure productive and therapeutic outcomes.

The growth and development of a group is directly related to the involvement of the members, which in turn has a direct bearing on the degree of cohesiveness that will develop in the group. Both involvement and cohesion bring members closer together and are therefore desired factors in and of themselves as well as being factors that contribute to the overall productivity of the group.

CHAPTER 4

Theoretical Approaches

A thought is often original though you have uttered it a hundred times.
— OLIVER WENDELL HOLMES

During the 1960s and 1970s the encounter (or sensitivity) group movement, with all its attendant controversies, was an umbrella term for the various approaches to personal growth (Posthuma & Posthuma, 1973). More recently, groups have become more individualized and have acquired specific labels denoting what they are about. For example, a person is now able to join a group for assertiveness training, time management, relaxation, or stress management, to name only a few. Contributing to the proliferation of personal growth groups was the expansion of theoretical approaches in group therapy (Ruitenbeek, 1970). Table 4-1 presents a concise comparative overview of selected theoretical approaches. Only four of these approaches are briefly reviewed here as it is anticipated that the reader will already be familiar with this information or can access it from other sources.

CLIENT-CENTERED THERAPY

Client-centered therapy was developed from the theories of self-actualization, which re-emerged in the mid-twentieth century, and stems primarily from the work of Carl Rogers (Geller, 1982). It is also known as nondirective or person-centered therapy. As the name implies, the client or individual is the central figure in this form of therapy. The key factor is the belief that the individual can be trusted to take responsibility for his own life without the direct intervention of a therapist (Ginsberg, 1984). Rogers emphasized the need for an open, honest, caring, accepting and nonjudgmental attitude on the part of the therapist. He believes that the key to a successful therapeutic outcome was the quality of the client-therapist relationship. In explaining the therapeutic relationship and his goals as a therapist he says, "To be a companion to my client as he or she explores the hidden mysteries of the inner life and to view that inner life as an acceptable part of reality — these are two of my chief goals in being a therapist" (Rogers, 1985, p. 43). He maintained that the three conditions necessary for a growth-promoting therapeutic climate were (1) genuineness and realness, (2) acceptance, caring, or confirming, and (3) empathy or understanding (Meador & Rogers, 1979).

This approach is particularly effective when used by a leader-therapist in a small group. Because of its nondirective aspects the group-centered approach allows the leader to do less "leading" with the result being increased participation by the group members. Rogers (1951) describes five distinctive functions carried out by the group-centered leader: (1) conveying warmth and empathy, (2) attending to others, (3) understanding meanings and intents, (4) conveying acceptance, and (5) linking.

CONVEYING WARMTH AND EMPATHY

It is difficult to describe just how a leader behaves to convey warmth and empathy but it appears to be behaviors and attitudes which manifest them-

Table 4-1. COMPARATIVE GROUP APPROACHES

Approach	Leader behavior	Therapeutic focus	Leader-member Relationship	Contents
Client-centered	Nondirective, conveying warmth, empathy, acceptance; active listening, paraphrasing, linking	Subjective experiences somewhat intrapsychic	Warm, open, positive, friendly, companionable	Anxieties, feelings, relationships, personal experiences
Behavioral	Reinforcing, modeling, limit setting	Specific behaviors	Contracting, businesslike, straightforward	Symptoms, anxieties, problems, overt behaviors, rehearsal for new behaviors
Psychoanalytic	Nondirective, passive, interpreting, probing	Intrapsychic events	Vague, changeable, spontaneous, health professional–client	Symptoms, life events, free association
Reality	Direct, limit setting, matter-of-fact, confrontive	Reality of events and existence	Problem solving, teacher–learner	Relationships, responsibility, fulfilling needs

Source: Adapted from J. L. Shapiro (1978). *Methods of group psychotherapy: A tradition of innovation.* Itasea, IL: F. E. Peacock.

selves in the leader's facial expressions, gestures, and speech. This basic manner in how the leader comes across is of utmost importance in creating a nonthreatening, accepting atmosphere. Rogers (1951) believes that the overall emotional tone of any group is greatly affected by the degree of warmth and empathy displayed by the leader. When group members identify with the leader they often internalize the same attitudes and behaviors that the leader displays. This means that group members will gradually become friendlier, warmer, and more empathic in their interactions with one another. Such conditions greatly enhance the quality and degree of communication in a group.

ATTENDING TO OTHERS

Most group members do not naturally possess effective listening skills. They find the act of listening attentively to another person a difficult task. This lack of skill emanates from a life's experience of focusing and working hard on our verbal expressions while, for the most part, ignoring our receptive abilities (Trotzer, 1977). Instead of attending, members are thinking ahead and formulating their responses or additional input. It is a common occurrence in groups for several members to successively bring up different points or ideas, none of which relate to the others. In such instances it is clear that the members are not attending to what others are saying. This lack of attention from others can cause some members to withdraw and refrain from participating because they sense their contributions are not being heard or welcomed (Rogers, 1951). The group-centered leader, by virtue of not needing to present or force her own views, is free to listen attentively to the contributions of each group member. The possession of the ability to closely attend to members is considered a primary skill of the group-centered leader. Trotzer expands this consideration by believing active listening to be the primary reaction skill for *all* group leaders and believes this is the behavior that conveys acceptance, respect, caring, and empathic understanding to the group members. These messages will not be conveyed if the leader-therapist is thinking:

- Are the members doing what I want them to do?
- I don't think what he said is true.
- I wonder if they like me?
- How can I get Mary involved?
- That is not important.

Given that active listening is a crucial interactive skill, then the question becomes, "How do you convey the message that you are really attending to what another is saying?" Such cues as looking directly at the person, nodding the head and offering some uh-huh's are helpful but one can do these and still not be listening. There are people who are very good at appearing attentive while their thoughts are miles away. However, if the listener reflects what has been said, then the speaker knows that he has been listened to. On receiving such undivided attention the member feels respected because he feels his contribution was received and is worthwhile. Leaders using a group-centered approach frequently begin their responses with phrases similar to:

> You are saying . . .
> You feel . . .
> If I understand you correctly . . .
> I gather that you mean . . .
> I'm not sure I follow you, but is it that . . .
> Let's see if I really understand that . . .

Gradually group members pick up this ability to attend by checking for understanding and meaning in what has been said by others. It can be very helpful in promoting interaction when members assume some of the responsibility for listening to others in this way. In terms of process, this involvement of the members is important as it allows the leader to relinquish parts of the leadership role and avoid the development of one-to-one dialogues with members. Passing on the skills of attending and reflecting to the members is thought to be a distinctive contribution, unique to group-centered leaders.

UNDERSTANDING MEANINGS AND INTENTS

As important as listening and reflecting are, these skills are not enough if people do not say what they mean, as is often the case. The leader then must try to bring out the "secret intent" of what has been said. By paraphrasing what the member has said the leader may help the member realize what he "really means."

Joe: I think we should end group early today. I'm tired.

Leader-therapist: You're feeling too tired to stay with us any longer.

Joe: Well I don't know if I'm tired or bored.

Leader-therapist: You don't know if you're really tired or just tired of what's going on.

Joe: Yeah, we haven't been talking about anything important.

Leader-therapist: So, the last little while has been pretty uninteresting for you.

Joe: Yeah, it was better in the last group when we talked about things that make us angry.

Leader-therapist: So, that discussion was more helpful to you. Let's see how the others feel about that.

From this exchange it appears that Joe did not really want to leave the group but rather wanted to talk about something else — perhaps more about anger.

Joe may not have realized this initially and thus could not say this outright. He was only aware of the fact that he did not like what was going on. The leader, through paraphrasing, enabled Joe to grapple with and then finally identify what actually promoted his statement. If the leader, in response to Joe's first statement. "I think we should end the group early today. I'm tired," had said something like, "It's only 15 more minutes, I think you should try and stay," then Joe is cut off. As a result, he may feel reprimanded and withdraw even further. When the leader-therapist uses paraphrasing to help Joe clarify his feelings, Joe feels accepted and encouraged to continue. Joe is finally able to express the real meaning and intent behind his desire to end the group.

CONVEYING ACCEPTANCE

In client-centered therapy, the therapist conveys complete acceptance of the client, and so must the group-centered leader-therapist convey acceptance of the individual members and the group. She must accept the group as it is at the moment. She must "convey a genuine acceptance of what the group members wish to discuss, what they decide to do and how they plan to do it" (Rogers, 1951, p. 355). This is not to say that the leader must be accepting if the members behave in ways that are malevolent or destructive and therefore totally unacceptable to the leader. In fact the group-centered leader is accepting "within limits" and these limits will depend on the boundaries of human decency, the structure and standards of the facility, and the values of the leader. However, because of the group-centered leader's belief in the abilities of the group members, she sets fewer limits than a leader who believes that she must tightly control the group. Group members who experience acceptance from the leader are likely to become more accepting and tolerant of their fellow group members. This accepting environment creates trust among members and promotes the sharing and exchange of genuine thoughts and sincere feelings in the group.

LINKING

The act of connecting the meaning of what one group member says to the meaning of what another member says is called linking. This skill depends largely on the insightfulness of the leader in ferreting out common themes or feelings from what different members say (Corey & Corey, 1982). To describe linking, Rogers (1951) uses the analogy of raindrops falling on a windowpane. Each raindrop represents a contribution by a group member and just as a raindrop forms a course of its own down the windowpane, so may each member's input stand alone. However, by using one's finger one can link up one raindrop's flow with that of another one, creating an enlarged raindrop which may or may not find a new course. The group-oriented leader can, in a similar fashion, link the thoughts of one member to those of another and as this process flourishes, the discussion gains strength and meaning as new contributions are linked in. For example, if Mary is sharing the despair she feels since her husband left her, the group-oriented leader could comment that her sense of loss and abandonment might be similar to the feelings experienced by Jim when his boss fired him or the way Anne felt when her parents asked her to move out. Linking in this way can facilitate interaction, sharing, and understanding among members. Sometimes the commonality of contributions is hidden and the leader-therapist, by clarifying the meaning of a comment, can facilitate the linking of ideas and promote a more encompassing discussion.

BEHAVIOR THERAPY

Within the behavior therapy approach there are a variety of procedures but the general goal of behavior therapy, "to create new conditions for learning" (Corey, 1982, p. 144), is common to all of them. The rationale that all behavior is learned and hence can be unlearned or replaced by new "learned" behavior is fundamental to behavior therapy. The basic constructs of reinforcement and extinction are among those most widely understood and universally applied (Waldinger. 1986). When working individually with clients, occupational therapists frequently employ tactics based on these two constructs. Therapists who praise a client's particular behavior ("It's nice to see you smiling this morning, Bob") know the value of reinforcement in encouraging a client to continue or repeat his effort. They also know that if they consistently ignore undesirable behavior, there is a good possibility that the behavior will eventually disappear.

These two constructs of behavior therapy, when employed in a small group setting, can be equally if not more effective than when used individually. In a group there is the opportunity for reinforcement to come not only from the leader-therapist but from the other group members as well. Such "multiple" reinforcement naturally carries a stronger message and therefore increases the impact of the message and the likelihood that change will occur. The same holds true for attempts at eliminating unacceptable behaviors. If the leader-therapist ignores a certain behavior exhibited by a member, the group members are likely to follow this example and ignore the member's behavior as well. The individual, feeling ignored by both members and the leader-therapist, may abandon his unacceptable behavior to regain a sense of acceptance.

Methods of behavior therapy that are particularly effective in advancing therapeutic outcomes in a group are contracting, cognitive restructuring, and modeling. Contracting, or drawing up an agreement with another person, can be an effective way to help clients who are having problems with some or all parts of the group experience. For example, an apathetic client may be experiencing difficulties such as getting to group on time, speaking in group, or staying for the specified period of time. If the member's lateness is especially disruptive the leader-therapist may initiate the formulation of a contract between the member and the group. Following a discussion of the problem, including how his tardiness affects the leader-therapist, other group members, and even the individual himself, an oral (or written) contract is suggested. The contract, which will contain behavioral objectives dealing with punctuality, will be an agreement between the tardy member and the total group. Through this contract, the member is actually saying "I will try to change," and the group is saying, "We want you to change and we want to help you to be successful in changing." This encouragement can be a powerful asset to the member and promotes a more supportive environment that is conducive to change. Because the contract creates a formal approach to the specified behavior it encourages all involved to examine the situation objectively and deal with it more constructively. In future, when the member arrives on time, not only will the successful behavior be lauded by the group but the successful adherence to the contract will also be recognized. Because the group now has a vested interest, when the member is once again late the group's response is more apt to be exploratory ("What happened?" "How can we help?") than hostile, as in the angry looks and comments ("You're late again") of before. In essence, with a contract you have two parties working toward change instead of just one.

Cognitive restructuring, which is rooted in Albert Ellis's rationale-emotive therapy, has more recently been linked with the treatment of depression (Beck, 1967, 1976). Simply put, cognitive restructuring means changing one's thoughts. Grieger and Boyd (1980) refer to this technique as "disputing irrational beliefs" (p. 130). It is rooted in the assumption that one's feelings and behaviors are directed by one's thinking and that distortions in the thinking process can cause negative emotions (depression) and maladaptive behaviors. Therapists of all disciplines are aware of how the I-can't-do-anything self-concept can affect a person's self-esteem, resulting in that person feeling "I am no good." Poor self-concept and low self-esteem are probably two of the most frequently used descriptors of persons suffering from emotional illness.

For decades, occupational therapists have been facilitating success experiences for their clients in order to increase their clients' self-esteem (Allen, 1985). In addition, occupational therapists are skilled in dealing with the problem areas that the techniques of cognitive behavior therapy focus on (i.e., interpersonal skills, problem solving, and self-management) (Johnston, 1987). Because occupational therapy is an activity-based treatment medium it affords ongoing opportunities to employ cognitive change methods. Whether in individual or group therapy, clients are most often involved in "doing." Even the smallest successes and accomplishments can be used to demonstrate the fallacies inherent in their automatic "can't-do" cognitions. All therapists have had clients who have automatic thoughts of "I'm stupid," or "This is stupid," which hamper their total approach to life. Changing these thinking patterns is a difficult first step in building confidence and capability. Haaga and Davison (1986) describe the need to go beyond modifying these automatic thoughts to determining the themes of the underlying dysfunctional assumptions and then modifying them. For example, the theme of the underlying dysfunctional assumption for the automatic thoughts focused on stupidity may be one of competence. So, by ensuring successful task experiences, the therapist can present a case for competent behaviors. Through discussion of the client's abilities she can help him become aware of how the shoulds ("I *should* be able to do it"), the musts ("I *must* do it perfectly"), and the have-tos ("I *have to* do it right") dominate his thinking and give rise to his distorted assumption of personal stupidity.

Using the same approach in a group the leader-therapist would select a task or activity that the group can successfully accomplish in order to promote thoughts of competence. While the members are involved in the activity she has the opportunity to point out negative thinking by the members and encourage them to watch for negative self-statements in one another. By helping members to become aware of distortions in their thinking patterns and the resultant faulty inferences they make, the leader-therapist can, along with the other members, assist a client in restructuring his thinking, practice new cognitions, and thus change the way he views himself. This process is depicted in Figure 4-1. Cognitive restructuring is useful in dealing with a wide variety of dysfunctional thoughts. For example, a description of how an occupational therapist could use this technique in helping a client control his stress and any subsequent feelings of anger is outlined by Taylor (1988).

Figure 4-1. Process of cognitive restructuring. (Source: Modified from S. D. Rose, Group methods. In F. H. Kanfer and A. P. Goldstein (Eds.), *Helping people change: A textbook of methods.* Elmsford, NY: Pergamon, 1986, pp. 437–469.)

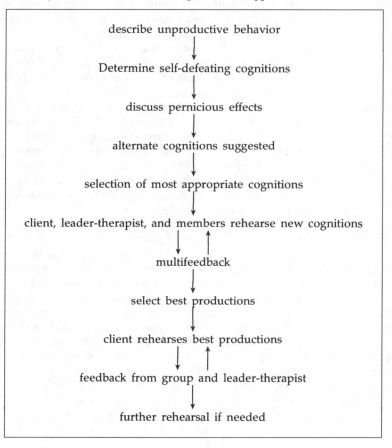

Small groups particularly lend themselves to the method of behavior therapy known as modeling. Trotzer (1977) points out that leaders serve as models whether they choose to or not and so should take advantage of opportunities to model desired group behaviors. Three major effects of modeling influences are described by Bandura (1971, p. 656). The first, the "observational learning effect," occurs when the observer reproduces a behavior that is exhibited by someone else (known as the model) but that was previously unknown and therefore new to the observer. This effect could be exemplified by a group member learning to express his feelings effectively when before he was unable to do so. A second effect of modeling is the decrease or increase of inhibitions of responses that already are part of the observer's behavioral repertoire. Such changes in inhibition are known as "inhibitory effects" and "disinhibitory effects" and are the result of observing positive or negative responses to the identified behavior in others. For example, if the observer, Bill, notices that whenever John swears he is cut off or completely ignored by the other members, then Bill is likely to curb or inhibit his own swearing. A third effect of modeling is known as "response facilitation effects" and this is the encouragement felt by the observer to repeat behaviors that are already familiar and present because they appear to be socially acceptable. A situation might be one where a member, John, who is tentative about expressing his feelings, sees that another member receives support and encouragement for saying how he feels. Observing this accepting and positive reaction by the members encourages John to express his own feelings more often.

With several individuals constituting a group, each member can observe a variety of behaviors as they are displayed by fellow members. This gives the members examples of alternative ways of behaving. Positive behaviors can be pointed out by the leader-therapist. For example, "Ann, I liked the way you accepted Mary's feedback," is an indicator that Ann's behavior was appropriate. Since all members are able to observe Ann's behavior it is possible for them to model that behavior in future similar situations. Of this component of modeling Bandura (1971) says that "when positive incentives are introduced, observational learning is promptly translated into action" (p. 658). Because of the significance of the leadership role a leader-therapist can have a strong influence on the behavior of group members through modeling desired behavior. The strength of this influence should always be kept in mind, as members are as apt to model "poor" behaviors as they are to model "good" behaviors. For instance, if the leader consistently arrives late to group she is likely to find that very soon the members will do likewise.

A leader-therapist employing a behavioral approach in a group may use several of the methods ascribed to classical behavior therapy. Used, even briefly, to deal with specific behavior problems, these procedures can be effective (Smith, Wood, & Smale, 1980).

PSYCHOANALYTIC THERAPY

Psychoanalytic group therapy is carried out by psychoanalysts who bring to the group the classical methods used in individual psychoanalysis. Although many of the methods of probing the unconscious that are central to psychoanalytic therapy are not appropriate for use by the majority of group leaders, some of the techniques and concepts can be valuable. Free association, a central technique in psychoanalytic therapy, can be a useful technique to apply in a group setting. In one-to-one therapy free association occurs when the client is instructed to "say whatever comes into your mind" (Corey, 1982, p. 23). These associations are believed to lead to the unconscious wishes, fantasies, conflicts, and motivations of the analysand. When transferred to a group setting, free association can be translated into "speak what's on your minds at any time" (Shapiro, 1978, p. 45). Giving a group this message, with its inherent freedom, can be very useful. It is a means of taking the pulse of the group, of finding out what members are thinking and feeling, what the issues are, and if they are shared. Instead of members feeling confined or inhibited in what they contribute, they feel more inclined to react or respond spontaneously, and in this way the free association is for the whole group. From this input the leader is able to get a sense of each individual, of the group as a whole, and of how they, the members, interrelate.

Another basic technique of psychoanalytic therapy that is useful in a group setting is interpretation, although the kind of interpretation that is appropriate in a group setting differs from that employed in classical analysis. It is important, when using the technique of interpretation in a group, to check for accuracy. Laying an interpretation on a group in a this-is-what-is-going-on manner without checking the validity of the interpretation or soliciting feedback can do more harm than good. It is best, if you are going to interpret, to do so in a speculative way ("You are all so quiet today. I'm wondering if you are a little angry that I was away last week?"), or to offer an individual interpretation ("Kathy, you seem to avoid talking with Jim. Do you think that could be related to the fact that he is about the age of your father?"). Interpretations can be effective catalysts to discussion and may prompt members to examine and think about their feelings and behaviors.

To expand on the cautionary note mentioned earlier, if used inappropriately interpretations can be offputting to some members. Interpreting behaviors or what individuals say can bring about defensiveness and cause some members to "clam up." They may feel threatened and angry at the leader-therapist for "reading things" into what they say and for trying to "psych them out." Once an interpretation has been rejected by a member it is best to let it go and try to make your point later or in some other way. Another hazard that can be encountered when making interpretations is the risk of encouraging an extended therapeutic interaction between the leader-therapist and one member (Yalom, 1970). Once an interpretation has been made, the leader-therapist is committed to working with the individual until a comfortable degree of understanding and acceptance has been reached. This working-through process often excludes the other group members and consequently may engender resentment toward both the leader-therapist and the identified member.

A knowledge and understanding of ego–defense mechanisms can help a leader-therapist recognize and analyze behaviors and dynamics that are present in the group as they occur. In referring to counselors in general, Corey (1982) says that "they can learn a great deal about the therapeutic process by becoming familiar with the concepts and techniques of the analytic approach" (p. 27). The same can be said about leader-therapists. Having an understanding of analytic constructs such as denial, avoidance, acting out, and resistance can be facilitative in learning about and understanding group process.

REALITY THERAPY

Whether or not you believe in the existence of mental illness, which William Glasser, founder of reality therapy, does not, the techniques of this approach are well suited to brief intervention situations. Because it is considered to be a short-term therapeutic method it lends itself to the process of therapy carried out in many small group settings. The functional, practical aspects of reality therapy make it an attractive and comfortable approach to therapy for occupational therapists. On examining the major techniques and procedures of reality therapy, one immediately sees the similarities between these procedures and some methods frequently used by occupational therapists:

1. Engage in role playing with the client.
2. Use humor.
3. Confront the client and do not allow any excuses.
4. Help the client to formulate specific plans for action.
5. Serve as a role model and teacher.
6. Set definite limits and structure the therapy situation.
7. Use "verbal shock therapy" or appropriate sarcasm to confront the client with his unrealistic behaviour.
8. Get involved with the client in his or her search for more effective living (Corey, 1982, p. 192).

Glasser (1965) maintains that all patients, no matter how severe their psychiatric problem, have the common characteristic of denying the reality of the world around them. He says patients deny reality because for them the real world has become a painful place from which they would like to escape. Patients may try to escape through psychotic or acting-out behavior, through physical illness, or suicide. Glasser therefore contends that the necessary therapy is one that would lead patients back to the realities of life.

According to the rationale of reality therapy the reason that patients reach the point of denying reality is because their needs are not being met. Glasser (1965) believes that everyone has two basic psychological needs that must be fulfilled in order for the person to be considered psychologically healthy: (1) the need to love and be loved, and (2) the need to feel that we are worthwhile to ourselves and others (p. 9).

Although everyone has these two basic needs, individuals differ in their abilities and resources to fulfill them. Those who are unable to fulfill these needs adequately may manifest problems and require help. To attain psychological well-being the most crucial factor is for a person to love and care for someone and be loved and cared for in return. Based on this premise, the aim of reality therapy is to help people regain involvement with others in order to give and receive love. The key concept in helping people is to motivate them to take responsibility for achieving this for themselves. A basic tenet of reality therapy is that patients are irresponsible and therefore they must learn to be responsible and work toward fulfilling their own needs. The optimal time to learn responsibility is when one is a child, but if it is not learned during childhood then it must be learned later on in life. From a reality therapist's point of view, the complete process of a person becoming dysfunctional and then gaining psychological health is as follows:

- Person does not love and is not loved
- Person does not feel worthwhile to himself or to others
- Needs are not met
- Person becomes irresponsible by giving up trying to meet his needs
- Psychological problems
- Person enters therapy
- Person is involved in relationship with therapist
- Person cares for and is cared for by therapist
- Person begins to feel worthwhile
- Person takes responsibility for fulfilling his needs
- Person fulfills his needs
- Psychological health

In reality therapy this process of gaining psychological health is based on eight principles (Glasser & Zunin, 1979). First, the therapist must be personal and warm in the therapeutic relationship and convey caring for the client. This has the purpose of showing the client that there is more to life than symptoms, misery, and irresponsibility. The circular interrelationship between feelings and doing is recognized, but the emphasis is placed on "doing" rather than on "feeling." So clients are encouraged to "do" better in order to "feel" better. Thirdly, reality therapy focuses on the present rather than on the past. It deals more with the results of behavior than with the causes of behavior. Value judgment is the fourth principle and clients are expected to make value judgments about their behaviors. The clients must decide whether their behavior, in each instance, could be considered responsible behavior. These judgments must be made not only in the context of the client himself, but also in view of the effect of the behaviors on those around him. The principle of planning is to help the client make specific plans to change behaviors that precipitate failure into behaviors likely to bring about success. It is suggested that such plans be put in writing, perhaps in the form of a contract.

The sixth principle, commitment, is considered by Glasser and Zunin to be the keystone of reality therapy. They believe that clients with "failure identities" have great difficulty committing themselves. Such persons may make their first commitment to the therapist ("I'll do this for *you*"), which is believed to be a first and positive step. It is thought that keeping commitments to others gives the individual a feeling of success and helps him achieve a "successful identity." Reality therapists do not accept excuses for failure nor do they dwell on the reasons for failure. They accept the situation and move forward ("Let's make a new plan" or "When are you going to do . . . ?"). Lastly, the reality therapist does not punish. Punishment is seen as a reinforcement of "failure identity" and therefore has no place in treatment. Therapists are cautioned to avoid any critical comments that can be construed as punishment by the client. The embodiment of these principles enables the therapist to help the client achieve psychological health through gaining a positive identity.

Whether you accept Glasser's blanket diagnosis of "irresponsibility" for all psychological problems or not, the practice of helping patients to become more responsible is a healthy one, and one used by most group leaders. Some ways in which leaders can and do help members to act responsibly are: (a) requiring members to be on time, (b) requesting members to inform the leader-therapist of any expected absence or late arrival, (c) giving members opportunities for decision making about the group's activities or discussion topics, (d) making it the responsibility of the members to get what they want from the group, (e) asking members to speak directly *to* one another and not *about* one another, and (f) reminding members that they are each responsible for their own behaviors, feelings, and any inferences they make. This last practice is an especially important one. Irresponsible persons tend to say things like "he made me so angry," or "she hurt my feelings," or "see what you made me do." By pointing out to members that they chose to feel angry or hurt or to do what they did is a way of helping them accept responsibility for the way they are and persuading them that if they want things to be different they have to bring about the change themselves.

SUMMARY

The four theoretical approaches presented here are by no means the only ones that a leader-therapist should draw from. They have been selected because they each view human behavior from a somewhat different perspective and each encompasses corresponding methods and techniques for altering behavior. As a leader-therapist you may find it most comfortable and productive to function within one framework only in your leadership role. However, it is more likely that on becoming familiar with several theoretical conceptualizations you will find an eclectic approach to be most facilitative. In this way you have more alternatives, techniques, and methods with which to respond to the dynamics as they unfold in your group. There are some settings where the theoretical approach of all professionals is dictated by the director or team. In such cases it is imperative that you feel comfortable in embracing the required approach. If not, you will find yourself constantly in conflict and at odds with the goals and premises of your coworkers. Of course, if you are feeling particularly dedicated, strong, and courageous, there is always the possibility of changing the beliefs and designated approach of your colleagues, but such endeavors are not for the faint-hearted.

To summarize the approaches presented here, the beliefs from which a client-centered therapist works are genuineness, acceptance, and empathy. Through careful attending and listening the therapist is able to convey caring and understanding and establish a warm therapeutic relationship with the client. The basic constructs of behavior therapy, reinforcement and extinction, underlie the useful therapeutic methods of contracting, cognitive restructuring, and modeling, which can be very productive techniques in group work. While the main thrust of psychoanalytic therapy, probing the unconscious, may not be appropriate in the classical sense for task groups, the attendant techniques of free association, interpretation, and an understanding of ego-defense mechanisms can be very useful. The eight principles of reality therapy, warmth, doing, dealing with the present, value judgments, planning, commitment, nonpunishing attitudes, and de-emphasizing failure, all help clients to move toward reality and away from dysfunction.

The reader will want to further explore those theoretical approaches of particular interest and investigate other theoretical approaches to develop a personal, comfortable, and effective style of leadership.

CHAPTER 5

Leadership

> *Who shall lead and who shall follow has often been of greater significance than where we shall go.*
> — EDWARD SAMPSON AND MARYA MARTHAS

People have been fascinated for centuries by the phenomenon of leadership. Perceived by some as the power of one person over others, the far-reaching effects of leadership concern every member of society (C. A. Gibb, 1969a, p. 9). Bass (1981) reflects that "the ancient art" of studying leadership is evident in the classical literature of the Greeks, Egyptians, and Chinese. The literature abounds with descriptions, theories, research, and discussions of what is meant by leadership and what exactly constitutes a leader. The very breadth of the topic defies a single, short, concise definition, although Cunningham and Carol (1986) make the effort with "leadership is the exercise of influence" (p. 73).

Influential leaders from the past in the areas of politics, religion, the military, and sports have been recognized and discussed as a means to understanding the concept of leadership. Leadership has been examined as it pertains to the leading of a country, a movement, a political group, a profession, a faith, a corporation, a business, a social group, and the present focus, a therapeutic group. In discussing the role of the leader in any group, Johnson and Johnson (1982) expand on the concept of influence: "A leader may be defined as a group member who exerts more influence on other members than they exert on him" (p. 49). In keeping with the notion of influence Sampson and Marthas (1977) describe a leader as a "person who is the most influential, who has the most power or the greatest ability to affect and alter the behavior of others" (p. 199).

In summary, leadership is assigned to or is assumed by persons who have exerted influence on others or are seen to have the ability to influence and thereby are viewed as potential leaders. In some instances a person can be pressed into the role of leader by other participants who do not wish to take on the role, but have a desire for the group to continue. In other cases persons may assume the leadership role because of their keen interest and involvement in a group's purpose or activities at a time when a leader is required. Whatever the case, any person who assumes a leadership role, be it of a Boy Scout troop, a volleyball team, or a political organization, is assuming a certain responsibility. Not always is the person aware of the degree of responsibility involved in the leadership role nor of the amount of work required to carry out the role. Some leaders function very successfully, others function well enough to hold the group together, while still others flounder and eventually pull out. Such a hit-and-miss process is not acceptable in a therapeutic situation. The leader-therapist must be knowledgeable, skilled, and personally masterful.

THEORIES OF LEADERSHIP

Theories of leadership abound. Some theories focus on factors relevant to the emergence of leadership, while others address the characteristics and consequences of leadership. From the former focus two theories have been selected for discussion here: the trait theory and the times theory. Subsequent chapters will explore characteristics and consequences of the leadership role.

TRAIT THEORY

The initial efforts to define and identify leaders concentrated on personality traits and characteristics (Schultz, 1986). Proponents of the trait or "great man" theory believed that leaders were born not made, discovered not developed. The basis of this belief was that persons rising to positions of leadership were born with certain characteristics or traits that enabled them to achieve their status. Aristole is credited with being one of the earliest proponents of this theory of leadership by saying, "From the moment of their birth, some are marked for subjugation and others for command" (Johnson & Johnson, 1982, p. 40).

Countless investigative studies have been done to determine what personality characteristics are conducive to an effective leader role (Jennings, 1960). Unfortunately (or fortunately, depending on your point of view!) the results were rarely found to agree on what were the essential characteristics (Spotts, 1969). Most studies have examined the characteristics or traits of persons established as leaders in social milieus such as the military, political, and business domains. Many of the trait studies have looked at leadership retrospectively, that is, they have studied individuals who are in leadership positions and from analyzing their attributes have identified common personality characteristics. It was then assumed that these common characteristics were the basic inborn qualities that produced a successful leader. Results were inconclusive in that individual studies demonstrated a great variety of personality traits that correlated with successful leadership roles (Latham, 1987). Such studies also made the point that not all persons with the same traits prove to be successful leaders.

Following an extensive survey of the literature on personality factors associated with leadership, Stogdill (1969) concluded that leadership was not merely the possession of a combination of certain personality characteristics. He believed, rather, that the important factor in successful leadership was the acquisition of those particular personality characteristics that facilitated relating to and working with members of the group for the achievement of common goals. He concluded that, in general, successful leaders were intelligent, insightful, and alert to the needs and motives of others. He also noted the importance of such traits as responsibility, initiative, persistence, and self-confidence. Johnson and Johnson (1982) summarize Stogdill's in-depth review of the literature: "Perhaps the safest conclusion to draw from the trait and personality studies of leadership is that individuals who have the energy, drive, self-confidence and determination to succeed will become leaders because they work hard to get the leadership positions" (p. 43).

TIMES THEORY

Proponents of the times or situation theory propose that leadership is a function of the particular social situation. A person may emerge as a successful leader in one situation but he may not be able to transfer this leadership role to another situation. In exploring the prediction of behavior from observed attitudes and personality traits, Sherman and Fazio (1983) emphasize the role that the situation plays in such predictions. They point out that people are not necessarily consistent in their behaviors and that in order to predict behavior one must consider both the individual and the situation. The situational leader is believed to have attitudes and skills that are required and peculiar to given situations and he will seek out such situations in order to express these qualities behaviorally. These unique qualities of the leader are seen to match the unique needs of the other members present in the situation. For example, a basketball team may thrust their team member who is most knowledgeable about the rules and requirements of the game into the team captain or leadership role. However, it is obvious that this same knowledge and the attendant skills will not be of value to the person if he chooses to play hockey instead.

The times theory is similar to the great man theory in that it assumes that certain characteristics or traits are prerequisites to any leadership role. However, it differs in that the characteristics required for leadership to develop in a given situation at a given time and place are unique to that situation. The great man theory attempts to define personality traits that are inherent and conducive to the role of the leader in general, whereas the times theory avers that the person most likely to assume a leadership role in any specific situation is the person most able to meet the needs of those involved.

THEORIES AND PRACTICE

The literature on leadership primarily addresses the leadership role and the functions of leaders in public domains. As mentioned in Chapter 1, sociologists played the prominent roles in the earliest look at processes that affected the masses. However by the late nineteenth century, sociologists were moving away from studying evolutionary change to studying directed change. Also at this time psychologists began to expand and broaden their study of the individual's involvement with others. According to Bonner (1959), these early investigations explored and demonstrated how certain persons could have influence on the performance of others. He points to a known fact today as being one of the most important findings of that era, "that a solitary individual and the same individual in a group are two different psychological structures" (p. 15). This deduction prompted much further research into the role of the individual in interaction with others. Naturally evolving from interest in interactive issues came absorption with and a plethora of investigations into the role of the leader. Resulting from and concurrent with these studies were the formulations of various theories of leadership.

Both the great man theory and the times theory have relevance for health professionals assuming leadership roles in small groups. Just as some persons assume the role of therapist with great skill and ease, so others assume the leadership role in small groups with the same degree of competence. The question is: can the essential skills for leadership be acquired or must individuals be genetically endowed with them? It is believed that these skills can be learned. It is also believed that although there are some basic skills required of all small group leaders, there are other skills that can be present in varying degrees with resultant successful leadership. We do not all have to be clones of the born leader!

The study of occupational therapy takes 3 to 4 years of professional study. During that time prospective occupational therapists learn a multitude of skills and methods of treatment. Some skills, such as seating and splinting, require physical dexterity and competence. Others are nonphysical but require keen mental processes to do the job, for example, interviewing and problem solving. Leadership skills, for the most part, fall into the latter category and can be learned in the same manner. Although each small group is a unique situation, there are some leadership skills that are necessary in each and every situation. There are other skills, though, that are more situation-specific and perhaps differentiate the effective leader from the less effective leader in a given situation.

THE LEADER-THERAPIST

Most occupational therapists must function as both individual therapists and group therapists. It is generally an established norm that any occupational therapist working in the area of mental health will run groups. Indeed, groups frequently form the greater part of the occupational therapy treatment program. Many therapists working in the areas of physical dysfunction, geriatrics, addiction, and forensic psychiatry also use groups in their treatment programs. Therefore it is imperative that the graduating occupational therapist have a thorough understanding of group process and be skilled and comfortable with the leader-therapist role. The term *leader-therapist* is used here to denote the dual role required by any professional leading a group. It is not enough to be purely a leader. One must function as a leader in a therapeutic manner. This means amalgamating the skills required in individual therapy with the skills required for effective leadership.

Therapists, and this refers to all health professionals who take on leadership roles in therapy groups, must have the education and training to function effectively in the role. As noted in this text there is a body of knowledge as well as various skills and techniques that the leader-therapist must be cognizant of and proficient in. The degree of small group leadership training incorporated in the curricula of the various professions varies widely, but competency should be the goal of all. Although occupational therapists and other health professionals function differently in their therapeutic leadership roles than do leaders in the public domain, it is important to the understanding of their leadership role to first understand some basic tenets about leadership in general.

Just as the professions vary in their approaches to therapy, so will leadership styles among members of any one profession vary. Leadership style refers to the way in which a person takes on the role of leader in a group. This style usually evolves from the person's basic personality and her typical manner of interacting with others. The style one assumes has an effect on the group and different styles evoke different processes and hence different outcomes. Sampson and Marthas (1981) believe there is a "self-fulfilling prophecy" inherent in the aspects and approach of a person's leadership style. Their premise is that "a particular leadership style gives rise to a particular membership style" (p. 205). For example, a leader whose assessment of human nature is that clients need to be led is likely to adopt a leadership style of directing and being in charge. This assessment stands to be confirmed by the members as they wait for direction, becoming more dependent than independent.

Leadership styles can be viewed along a continuum, from the position of responsibility for the group being assumed primarily by the leader to that of responsibility being appropriated by the members. This continuum was graphically outlined by Tannenbaum and Schmidt (1958) and is adapted for presentation in Figure 5-1.

It is useful for leaders to plot themselves periodically on this continuum as a means of assessing their leadership style. A therapist may not always utilize the same leadership style. A person may change her style in order to better respond to a situation or to a group's needs at a particular time. For example, with a newly formed group where the members have little idea of what is expected of them individually or of the group as a whole, the leader may decide it is appropriate and facilitative in this instance to be highly directive. With an ongoing group it may be the leader's decision to give the members more autonomy and allow them to function as independently as possible.

This need for flexibility is seen as a major problem with the style approach to understanding leadership. Johnson and Johnson (1982) emphasize the need to adjust leadership style to the situation. For example, in a situation where an urgent decision must be made, an autocratic leadership style would be most effective. In a different situation where input from the group members is desired to ensure that the decision made will be implemented, a democratic style would be more appropriate. A laissez-faire leadership style might be best if the members are committed to a plan, have the resources they need, and the abilities to proceed with the project on their own.

The different leadership styles are described separately here in order only to help clarify the differences. The intent is not to imply that one is better than the others or that there are inherent "good" and "bad" components, but only to show the variety of behaviors that are evident in and available to those in leadership roles. Each leader creates her own way of being in the role, by incorporating behaviors that feel the most comfortable and which prove to be the most efficient. A sensitive leader-therapist will combine whatever components of the three styles are needed to function effectively and carry out her leadership role at any given moment in the life of the group.

LEADERSHIP STYLES

The categories of leadership styles most often described in the literature are those defined in the classic studies by Lewin, Lippitt, and White (1939). They describe three styles: democratic, a member-centered problem solving style;

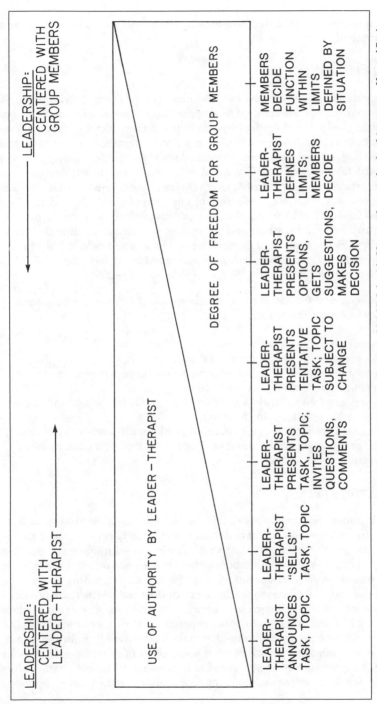

Figure 5-1. Leadership continuum. (Source: Modified from R. Tannenbaum and W. H. Schmidt, How to choose a leadership pattern. *Harvard Business Review*, 36, 95, 1958.)

autocratic, a leader-centered decision-making style; and laissez-faire, neither a leader nor member-centered style.

DEMOCRATIC STYLE

As mentioned, this style can best be described as a problem solving style. A leader employing a democratic style attempts to create a safe environment within which group members feel free to express their views, thoughts, and feelings without fear of being rejected or put down. Members are encouraged to be themselves, to deal with their diversities through problem solving, and to move toward taking responsibility for the direction and functioning of the group. The process may be lengthy, as it requires time to ensure that all ideas are considered and discussed, differing opinions are worked out, and conflicts are resolved in an effort to accomplish the mutual goals. It is an active process directed at involving all members and as much as possible at meeting the needs of all members. Some aspects of democratic style are noted below. The characteristics of the three leadership styles, as presented here, have been taken in part from a summary offered by Verba (1961, pp. 208–209)

1. All policies are matters of group discussion and decision, encouraged and assisted by the leader.
2. Leaders
   • guide rather than direct a group
   • are receptive to group members' suggestions
   • leave most of the decision making to the group members
   • may offer suggestions or alternatives
3. Members are free to work with whomever they choose and the division of tasks is left up to the group.
4. The leader is objective or fact-minded in his praise and criticism and tries to be a regular group member in spirit without doing too much of the work.

AUTOCRATIC STYLE

In the continuum of leadership styles laid out in Figure 5-1, the autocratic style is found at the extreme left of the continuum and centers on the leader-therapist rather than on the members. Autocratic leaders need to have control and be in charge. They *do to* group members rather than allow group members *to do* for themselves or *to do* in cooperation with the leader. According to Dimock (1985c), leaders whose style is to teach, direct, or dominate, lessen the possibilities and opportunities for the group to grow and develop. Autocratic leaders have a I-know-best attitude and do not encourage members to participate in the decision making process but rather tend to make all the decisions for the group. Members are frequently unaware of what is expected of them overall, of what the goals of the group are or what is going to happen next. The autocratic leader is not interested in the personal goals of group members but rather operates from personally designed goals for the whole group. Frequently such goals meet the personal needs of the leader. Alternative ideas are discouraged and discussion is kept to a minimum, to prevent bonding between members. In short, the leader runs the show and members do what they are told or asked to do. This does not mean that such leaders are necessarily harsh or hostile. In fact they can be very friendly as they persuade the group that they know what is best and what is the right way to do things. When members comply, the auto-cratic leader gives the individuals praise, which may appear generous but has the tendency to separate members and encourage competition for the leader's favor. J. R. Gibb (1969) believes that autocratic leaders generally assume that people cannot be trusted and he refers to this style as "defensive leadership." He describes such leaders as using persuasion and a reward system to control their members. Group goals are forgotten in attempts to gain recognition from the leader.

All this may seem to imply that the autocratic leader is a "bad" leader. This is not necessarily the case. As has been mentioned there are times in a group's life when it is appropriate for the leader to assume a more authoritarian stance in order that the group may move forward. One example is when the members of the group are very low-functioning and are therefore unable to show initiative, make decisions, or assume responsibilty. The main point to be cognizant of is that the person who tends to be autocratic in most of her daily interactions should be aware of the effects of carrying such personality traits over into her leadership role. The characteristics of an autocratic leader are:

1. All decisions and determination of policy are made by the leader.
2. Techniques and activity steps are directed by the leader one at a time so that future steps are always uncertain to a large degree.
3. The leader usually dictates the particular work task and work compan-ion of each member.
4. The leader tends to be "personal" in her praise and criticism of the work for each member, but remains aloof from active participation except when demonstrating.

Two other styles of leadership, bureaucratic and diplomatic, are discussed by Burgoon, Heston, and McCroskey (1974). Although they pertain more to social groups than therapeutic groups they are worth noting. The bureaucratic leader is impersonal and rule-centered. He is interested in security, avoids communi-cation with his members, and demands loyalty. His relationship with the mem-bers is more official than personal, which in turn tends to precipitate apathy among group members. This style of leadership is similar to the "push" type of leadership delineated by Cooper and McGaugh(1969).

The diplomatic leader is described as Machiavellian because of her manipu-lative characteristics. She looks for personal gain in her leadership role and uses various tactics to achieve her desired ends. Although at times she may appear democratic in her manner of engaging the members, there is usually an underlying personal motivation.

LAISSEZ-FAIRE STYLE

The leader who adopts a laissez-faire style could best be described as a non-leader. As the French implies, this leader just "lets it be"; her nondirectiveness lets whatever will happen in the group happen. Goals are not established, the purpose of the group is not clearly explained, members are not encouraged by the leader to participate, decisions are not made, and the leader remains more or less removed from the whole process. There are times when untrained leaders fall into this style through lack of skill or knowledge of what to do. Other leaders adopt the style as a defense against telling others what to do or, as they perceive it, of being authoritarian. They believe the group members will rise to the occasion, take charge, and direct themselves. Unfortunately, what frequently occurs in such situations is that members flounder, feel frustrated, confused, and sometimes hostile, and generally are nonproductive. Occasionally a group member will emerge in a leadership role and attempt to organize the group. This can either offer the direction that the group needs or, conversely, it can increase the feelings of frustration in that a group member has to do the leader's job.

In a therapy group, since such a situation causes frustration and confusion, a laissez-faire leadership style often only serves to increase the anxiety level of the members, causing them to withdraw and feel resentful of the group experience. One might argue that such a situation is a way to assess how members handle anxiety and to find out which members, if any, attempt to take charge. However, it is felt that the same information can be obtained by less stressful means, without the risk of clients being totally turned off to further group experiences.

A laissez-faire style of leadership is not compatible with running a task group as the task itself lends some order and direction to the group. Since task groups are the forte of occupational therapy groups, it is less likely that occupational therapists will find this leadership style very productive or useful as a primary style. Having said this, a qualifying statement is necessary. There are times when the leader-therapist will assign a task or a problem to the group with the instructions that they are to work on it on their own. This format encourages the members to practice leadership, problem solving and decision-making skills, cooperative measures, and self-reliance. The process, observed by the leader-therapist and experienced by the members, is then discussed so the overall dynamics can be clarified and integrated. Aspects of the laissez-faire style are:

1. Complete freedom for individual or group decision making, with a minimum of leader participation.
2. Materials are supplied by the leader, who makes it clear that she will only supply information if asked. The leader takes no part in work or discussion.
3. Complete nonparticipation of the leader in determining tasks and companions.

4. The leader makes infrequent comments on member activities unless questioned, and makes no attempt to appraise or regulate the course of events.

The three leadership styles are formally depicted in Figure 5-2. As can be seen, in the democratic style the leader's direct interaction is with the group and the group is responsible for decisions. This differs from the autocratic leader where there is no link between the group and decision making. With this style all information must be processed through the leader, who with little interaction or discussion makes the decisions. The laissez-faire style represents very little involvement by the leader with either the group or the decision-making process, as the latter is primarily left to the group.

COMBINATION OF STYLES

Most group leaders operate primarily from one leadership style, which has as its basis the leader's own personality traits. A person of action who likes to get things done quickly and who has strong opinions about how things should be is more likely to adopt an autocratic leadership style than one who is more easygoing. A person who enjoys interacting and listening to the ideas of others, joining in a problem solving process and being part of a discussion, is prone to be a more democratic leader. An aversion to authority of any kind and a strong belief in the autonomy and rights of the individual are characteristics that would lead a person toward a laissez-faire style. As can be seen in examining these traits, positive aspects can be found in each, which can be used productively in combination.

Let us examine the situation where you, the leader-therapist, are beginning your first session with a new group of clients. You have chosen a consensus task as the activity for the session. Initially you introduce yourself and suggest, depending on whether members know one another or not, that the members also introduce themselves (autocratic). You might then ask if any members have any questions or anything they want to say before you begin the activity (democratic). You then describe the task, state the rules, explain how it is to be done, and give a time limit (autocratic). At this point you would again ask if there are any questions (democratic). During the task you might withdraw from participation and let the group function entirely on its own even responding to certain questions with "what do you think?," or "it's up to you" (laissez-faire). At the end of the stated time you terminate the task (autocratic) and move the group into a discussion of what happened during the activity and how members felt about the experience (democratic). Combining approaches in this way makes for a diverse and interesting leader. It can also be quite productive, as the group members feel some autonomy but are prodded to keep moving.

Having a clear understanding of the differences in the three leadership styles can be helpful in determining your own style. It can be informative to evaluate

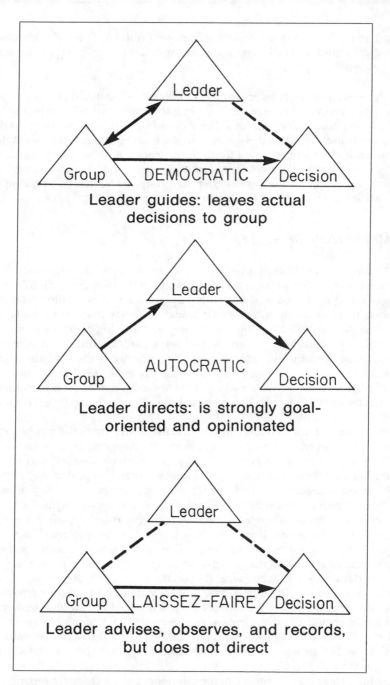

**Leader guides: leaves actual
decisions to group**

**Leader directs: is strongly goal-
oriented and opinionated**

**Leader advises, observes, and records,
but does not direct**

Figure 5-2. Three basic styles of leadership.

your personal characteristics and then relate and compare them to the leadership characteristics. As an example, you may realize that you are quite extroverted and a rather high-powered type of person. You like to make decisions and get things done. Knowing this you may conclude that your most natural way of operating in any group is to tend to take charge, organize, and prod members to action. You may conclude that your personality appears to embrace both democratic and autocratic traits, but few that could be considered laissez-faire.

An awareness of the styles can also add to your repertoire of leadership behaviors by stimulating alternative actions. Say a group is working intently on a consensus task but 5 or 10 minutes into the task, member A, appearing distressed, makes the following statement: "No one will listen to me." At this point it is important to set aside the task temporarily and facilitate within the group a discussion of member A's feelings. It is even possible that the task may be completely abandoned for that session in favor of continuing what has evolved into a very productive discussion. For some leaders it is very difficult to be this flexible. They feel a need to have the task completed and therefore will defer such a discussion or ignore the member's input until the task is finished. By the end of the task, however, the moment may be lost and member A or other group members may be resistant to discussing the issue. It is more difficult for members to recall feelings than to deal with them in the here and now. Discussing an issue in retrospect can lapse into a dialogue of, "You said," "No, I didn't," "Yes you did" — the sort of situation that is obviously unproductive. On the other hand, if the above discussion starts to meander off the topic or is resolved to what you believe to be (on checking) member A's and the group's satisfaction, then it is a good time to direct the members back to the task.

EFFECT OF LEADERSHIP STYLE ON GROUP MEMBERS

The behavior or style of the leader will have a direct effect on the behavior of group members (Sampson & Marthas, 1981). This is particularly true if the leader functions exclusively within one style of leadership. The behavior of group members as consequences of leadership style are known as membership styles and are presented below, based in part on those discussed by Sampson and Marthas (1981).

Democratic Style

1. Members are enthusiastic about the task or activity of the group, displaying a high degree of participation and involvement.
2. Members are motivated to complete the task and experience satisfaction from being part of a successful effort.
3. There is a strong sense of unity or we-ness among group members as they cooperate and work together. Members are accepting and caring of one another.

4. Members feel good about their own participation and encourage it in others.
5. Members display initiative and learn to assume responsibility for the functioning and progress of the group.

Autocratic Style

1. Members will be compliant in doing the task but will show little enthusiasm. Participation or involvement may appear forced or stilted.
2. Members can be productive in working on the task but feelings of satisfaction are absent due to resentments and anger toward the leader.
3. Cooperation is low and members may be irritable and blaming with one another.
4. Participation by members is dependent on prodding from the leader.
5. Members resist accepting responsibility, display little initiative, and are apathetic toward what happens in or to the group.

Laissez-faire Style

1. Members are confused and frustrated with the task due to lack of direction.
2. Productivity is low. Efforts at completing the task may be sloppy and inefficient.
3. Members are not unified and display little interest in working together.
4. Participation is uneven and unrelated to the participation of others.
5. Due to the confusion and frustration experienced by members with the purpose of the group, they tend to absolve themselves of responsibility for what happens.

It should be recognized that the member behaviors described here represent reactive responses to the leadership styles in their most classic and pure forms. Rarely does a leader-therapist perform "classically." These behaviors are more likely to be observed in combination.

Observing the behaviors of group members, especially over time, can sometimes be cause for an analysis of your behaviors as leader-therapist. If approached with a receptive mind this can be an enlightening process and may provoke you to adapt or make some definitive changes in your approach. Self-evaluations should be frequent and ongoing (and not only when there are problems) to prevent repetition, rigidity, and stagnation.

SUMMARY

Formulating your own leadership style is a very personal and individual process. Although new behaviors can and should be learned, attempting to function at complete odds with your basic personality set is unrealistic. Success comes when you can effectively incorporate your personal characteristics into the many facets and functions that form the composite of a leader-therapist's role. In this role you must direct, facilitate, observe, analyze, participate, listen, respond, organize, and remember that you are usually seen as an expert. Your success in these endeavors will be contributed to in part by your mix of personal characteristics (the great man theory) and in part by the situation, (the times theory).

Although, the three leadership styles, democratic, autocratic and laissez-faire, are presented separately, it is suggested that leader-therapists incorporate those behaviors from each style that they feel most comfortable with and which prove to be most productive at any given time in a particular group session. In a similar manner to selecting methods and techniques from various theoretical approaches, so do you select behavior from the different leadership styles. In general, you may adopt more behaviors from one style than from the others, but it is wise to be flexible and eclectic in your overall approach. You must also always keep in mind that your leadership style will have a direct influence on the behavior of the group members. It is a responsible and exciting role that is best carried out with sensitivity. Specific leadership skills and techniques are covered in the following chapters.

CHAPTER 6

The Leader-Therapist

> *The most effective leader is
> one who can create the
> conditions by which he
> will actually lose the
> leadership.*
> — *CARL ROGERS*

One of the expectations of therapeutic groups is that the members will be involved in ongoing self-evaluation to facilitate change in themselves. Leader-therapists should be involved in the same process. A group leader learns from each group experience, as do the members of the group, and consequently both are in a constant state of change. The leader-therapist needs to practice what all therapists preach: recognizing behaviors that need improvement is the first step toward positive change. Following each group session the leader-therapist will benefit from engaging in a self-analysis as well as an analysis of the group process. This self-analysis should focus on thoughts, feelings, and behaviors experienced and displayed during the session. The following attributes of leadership can serve as useful referents in guiding one's self-analysis.

ATTRIBUTES

An inherent difficulty in delineating the critical attributes of a leader-therapist is related to the wide variety of qualities and characteristics that contribute to effective leadership. In addition, the individual's personality, the purpose of the group, and the nature of the members all must be taken into consideration when identifying desired characteristics. The attributes selected for inclusion here are thought to be representative of basic qualities that seem to have a commonality among effective leaders.

SELF-CONFIDENCE

In any endeavor we function more productively if we have confidence in what we are doing. Corey, Corey, and Callanan, (1979) describe the most effective counselors as those who feel like "winners." Group members will be quick to pick up on lack of confidence in a leader and this may cause them to feel uneasy and wary of getting involved in the group. It is scary to take personal risks if you do not feel confident that the person in charge is capable and dependable. So a certain level of self-confidence demonstrated by the leader is necessary to inspire confidence in the group members (Kottler, 1983). By showing self-assurance, enthusiasm, and comfort in the situation you are more able to facilitate member participation and hence a productive group experience for all. Members' perceptions of an effective helper are formed from various indicators, one being "dynamism," which encompasses self-confidence and forcefulness. Research by Goldstein and Myers (1986) demonstrated that people are more attracted to high-status helpers or persons perceived to be experts than to those perceived to be lower-status helpers. Of four variables selected by Schultz (1986) as predictors of emergent leadership, "self-assured" was the only one related to personal style. The other three, "formulates goals," "gives directions," and "summarizes," were all communicative functions.

Naturally, one gains self-confidence in the leadership role with experience, but even as a novice leader-therapist it is important to impart the message of capability. The old adage, "you are what you feel," holds true. If you present in a positive manner, called "performance self-esteem" by Stake (1983), and believe that you are competent to run a productive group, then it is highly likely you will have a productive group. Kottler (1983) emphasizes this need for a "strong sense of mission" in the leader. To introduce a task or activity with "this experience can be very helpful," will produce a more positive response from the group members than will the hesitant "this might be useful, but I'm not sure."

In the same way that members do, the leader-therapist takes her own fears, needs, and anxieties into the group with her (Penland & Fine, 1974). She wonders, "Will the group be successful?," and worries, "Am I ready for this?" If she is able to move beyond these questions within herself to "hearing" these same questions in her group members, she will demonstrate sensitivity, awareness, and understanding. By doing this she will achieve a sense of mastery over her own anxieties, function more effectively, and present an aura of competence. Using each group as a learning experience will gradually but consistently build self-confidence in the role of leader-therapist.

RESPONSIBILITY

This attribute, which here embodies dependability, trustworthiness, and reliability, is an important one but a difficult one to explain. A leader-therapist can be seen to have dual responsibilities, one to the group and one to herself as a professional. The leader-therapist, usually the only staff member in the group, must assume full responsibility for handling the "happenings" in the group. Members of the group need to feel safe and know that they can depend on the leader-therapist to ensure their safety by having their best interests at heart. There must be trust that the leader-therapist will behave responsibly toward all members. Trotzer (1977) describes leader responsibility as being on a continuum. At one extreme the leader-therapist assumes full responsibility for all the "interactions and impact of the group," while at the other extreme, the responsibility is totally invested in the group, including the leader-therapist as an equal partner (p. 91). Most leader-therapists operate from the *middle* of the *continuum,* giving and taking responsibility in response to the needs and level of functioning of the group. Frequently the degree to which responsibility is assumed reflects the developmental level of the group. When the group is in a dependent phase the leader-therapist may accept more responsibility which she then gradually gives over to the group as it demonstrates more independence. This transition could even occur over the course of one session.

Sharing responsibilities can at times be part of the goals and functions of the group. During a task or activity the leader-therapist may encourage members to accept responsibility by asking, "Who would like to keep the list?," or, "Who will be responsible for announcing the time slots?" Responsibilities can extend outside the group as in, "Would someone set up the chairs for the next session?," and sometimes the group may be given total responsibility for organizing the task or activity for a session. Trust is an issue in terms of confidentiality. The leader-therapist must be honest and inform the members what the limits are for information remaining confidential to the group. A trustworthy leader does not tell a member she will keep certain information confidential but then report the information to her colleagues. However, a leader-therapist also has a responsibility to her team members and she must tread this line with care. To be responsible to both colleagues and group members it is best to be up front with the latter by telling them that what goes on in any group session is usually reported back to the team. Explain the importance of all team members having this information in order to optimize overall treatment and goal planning. By explaining this to the group members, they then know where they stand in terms of confidentiality and thus can choose what they wish to share in the group.

As for reliability and dependability, group members prefer a leader-therapist whom they can rely on to behave in a consistent manner from one session to another. They like a leader-therapist who is dependable, who arrives on time, who makes sure a suitable meeting room is available, and who has given some forethought to the session such as having a task prepared or the required materials available for a planned activity.

ATTENDING AND LISTENING

Although to some, listening may appear to be a leadership technique, it is included here because of its importance as a personal attribute. People who are good listeners by nature tend to make good leader-therapists. When asked why they joined a helping profession counselors often reply, "Well, I always have been a good listener." However, if you do not count listening or attending among your main strengths, do not despair for they are skills that can be acquired through practice and perseverance.

The leader-therapist role is an exacting one as you must be *tuned in* to all members of the group for the entire session. Sound exhausting? It can be. As a preparatory measure to this demanding experience it is energizing to "psych" yourself up to listen before entering the session. Being tuned in means not only listening to what each member says but listening to how they say what they say. It also means attending to all the nonverbal messages that members may be conveying. Frequently the latter are of more consequence than the former. Lakin (1983) recognizes that the demands of listening and attending to all the verbal and nonverbal communications occurring simultaneously among the group members is a major source of stress for group leaders.

The leader-therapist must listen very carefully and really hear what is being said in order to connect with group members. Another aspect of the leader-therapist's role is to encourage this listening behavior in others in the group to facilitate connections between the members. It is this linking that spawns the growth of trust, a condition crucial to the growth and development of a group. By listening and attending to members' responses a leader-therapist can tell if the members are actually listening to one another. The importance of their doing so can be emphasized by statements such as, "From what you replied I'm not sure you really heard what M. said," "What did you hear M. say?," or, "Can you repeat what M. just said?" Sometimes what you hear and what you see do not appear to be congruent. For example, a member may be telling you how happy he is and how well things are going for him, while all the time he is speaking he is looking anything but happy. In this instance attending gives you information that differs from that which you hear. To deal with the inconsistency you might say something like, "What I heard you say is . . . but it doesn't seem to fit with the sad look on your face." From these or similar interventions members receive the message that not only are you interested in what they have to say but also whether what they say is correctly understood by the other members.

There are many ways that both leader-therapists and members demonstrate a lack of listening and or attending:

- Lack of eye contact
- Interrupting
- Thinking of what to say next
- Talking too much
- Being off-topic
- Hearing what you want to hear

Effective listening requires concentration. It is better to listen and then take a few seconds to consider what members have said before you respond than to be thinking of your response while they are speaking. After all, you will not know what they have said until they have said it!

There are several different modes of listening (Purtilo, 1978), and the leader-therapist will engage in some modes more often than others. She will listen *attentively* when general information is being offered and her goal is to comprehend the whole picture. This level of listening is crucial to avoid missing small but important bits of information. Her listening can be *analytical* if she is looking for specific kinds of information. For example, the leader-therapist will be interested in discerning the problem areas of a new group member. In analyzing what she hears she is able to classify the problems into different categories, perhaps family, personal, work, or dependent-independent. Using *directed* listening the leader-therapist is attempting to answer a specific question. To use the previous example, at a later time the leader-therapist may hope to answer the question, "Does this client have any positive relationships within his family?" In this case her listening would be directed more toward comments he makes about his family than toward any other information he shares.

Leader-therapists often engage in *exploratory* listening, which indicates an interest in all aspects of the topic under discussion. In this instance they are keen to hear the thoughts and ideas of all the group members. Sometimes listening is *courteous* as in feeling obliged to listen. This could happen when a new group member, who has not yet grasped the purpose or norms of the group, expands on a there-and-then irrelevant experience. Under the circumstances it seems courteous to hear him through before going on to something more relevant. There are also inadvertent events that precipitate a leader-therapist listening *passively*, as when she hears people speaking just outside the group room. Her focus is on the group but because of the proximity of the voices she cannot avoid hearing them. This could also occur within the group if two members speak quietly as a dyad while another member is talking to the group as a whole. The leader-therapist will be passively hearing the dyad as she listens attentively to the speaking member. The last mode of listening is known as *appreciative*, which is the kind of listening one does for pleasure, such as listening to music or the sounds of the sea.

Listening, or what is heard, generates many feelings, thoughts, and behaviors in people. Barker, Wahlers, Cegala, and Kibler (1983) list five listening pitfalls to avoid in a group.

1. Getting overstimulated or emotionally involved.
2. Preparing to answer questions before fully understanding them
3. Tolerating or failing to adjust to distractions
4. Allowing emotionally laden words to interfere with listening
5. Permitting personal prejudices or deep-seated convictions to impair comprehension or understanding (p. 88)

OBJECTIVITY

As in all therapeutic roles it is imperative that the leader-therapist maintain a firm sense of objectivity. Rogers (1961) describes an "as if" quality in defining empathy that can be related to objectivity. He believes that individuals who respond *as if* they were the other person without losing their personal identity can be empathic while still retaining their objectivity. A leader-therapist must be able to think clearly and maintain an objective awareness of all the members, even when under pressure. To become subjectively immersed in the issues or problems of one member of the group is to be out of touch with the others. In addition, to experience this degree of subjective involvement is draining and depletes the energy required to deal with the other group members or the day's routine that follows. As leader-therapist you can be empathic but remain aware that the problem belongs to the other person and not to you. Leader-therapists must constantly monitor their own feelings and responses to ensure their objectivity. Indicators of nonobjective behaviors are (a) getting caught up in the content and forgetting about the process of the group, (b) experiencing overwhelming emotions, (c) assuming the roles of advice giver and problem solver, and (d) arguing.

An integral part of being objective is the ability to recognize the presence of transference and countertransference among your members and within yourself. Transference refers to the stimulation and emergence of suppressed or repressed feelings in a group member as a result of interacting with the leader-therapist or another group member (Kaplan & Sadock, 1985). As an example, a member may react angrily toward the leader-therapist because for him she stands for a significant person from his past, perhaps an authoritative or domineering mother. Because these experiences and attitudes differ for each member the reactions of the members to you will also be varied. It can be confusing to have some members react very positively to your participation while others seem quite resistive and negative. In leading a group you "can't please all of the people all of the time." It is important to help your members recognize any distorted perceptions they may have, such as your being all-knowing or your being vindictive, and to help them work through the feelings toward you that have been engendered by these distortions.

It can be more difficult to deal with countertransference. Since these feelings and reactions occur within you, the leader-therapist, a great deal of self-awareness is required for you to recognize the dynamics that are taking place (Sampson & Marthas, 1981). It is only too easy to be responsive to positives and accept accolades while becoming defensive in response to negatives or disagreement. The key is to try to maintain a critical awareness and sensitivity to all that is happening both in your group members and within yourself.

GENUINENESS

To be genuine implies that what you do and say is congruent with what is going on inside of you (Rogers, 1961). To be genuine as a leader-therapist is to behave without pretense. It means that you are sincere and you do not pretend to be that which you are not. You do not hide behind defenses or your leadership role but rather you are authentic and able to honestly share your thoughts and feelings with the group. It is even appropriate at times for the leader-therapist to share her own fears or anxieties with the group. This demonstrates to the group that being afraid and anxious is universal and that even you, the leader, experience these feelings (Derlega & Chaikin, 1975). By being genuine yourself you are more likely to elicit the same behavior in others and serve as a role model to encourage genuine behavior in your group members. Rogers cites the following characteristics as being essential to forming a therapeutic relationship: (1) congruence, or genuineness; (2) unconditional positive regard; and (3) accurate empathic understanding. Of these three he believes genuineness to be the most important.

EMPATHY AND CARING

In a recent survey of occupational therapy educators, the skill, "be empathic and genuine," was rated the most important of 32 skills and techniques judged to be relevant to a psychosocial occupational therapist (Barris & Kielhofner, 1986). The question then is, "How does one become empathic and genuine?"

While there is one school of thought suggesting that genetic factors may influence a person's ability to be empathic (Matthews, Batson, Horn, & Rosenman, 1981), others believe that the ability to be empathic can be learned and is part of the development of social skills (Yalom, 1983). A person displays empathy when she is able to understand and be sensitive to the feelings and experience of others, to "walk in their shoes" and understand their world. When group members experience empathic understanding from the leader-therapist or other members they are more likely to continue sharing and exploring because they feel understood and accepted. Goldstein and Myers (1986) view empathic responding as one of the crucial conditions in effecting client change.

At times it is difficult for a young leader-therapist to understand the feelings of a member because she has not yet lived the variety of life situations that come only with age and experience (Posthuma, 1976). However, one can still show empathic understanding by being sensitive to and responding to the feelings displayed: "I can see that it is upsetting for you to talk about what happened. It must be very painful." Such a response conveys caring, acceptance, and understanding. Compare it to this response: "I can see that you are upset but you will soon get over it." Responses such as the latter block members from sharing themselves further and prevent them from exploring their experience. Other responses that are nonempathic are critical judgments, blunt questions, telling others how they should or should not feel, being flippant, or ignoring a person and moving on to something else.

Empathy can be conveyed nonverbally as well. This can be done with an understanding or caring look, a smile, a touch of the hand, or an arm around the shoulder. Some therapists feel uncomfortable with touching, often because of being raised in our hands-off society, but if motivated to do so they can, with practice, become more comfortable as touchers (Posthuma, 1985).

While it may be that a person is able to feel truly empathic only with certain individuals, it is important to be compassionate to all. To be compassionate is to respect and care about others, to be sensitive to their feelings and to have a deep concern for their welfare. A compassionate leader-therapist offers herself selflessly in the spirit of helping and professionalism.

WARMTH

This attribute is noted separately due to its importance, although it is recognized that empathy and caring usually convey a feeling of warmth. These and other helping procedures can, however, be technically correct but when carried out without warmth they are "therapeutically impotent" (Goldstein & Myers, 1986). Because warmth in the therapist begets warmth in the client, a reciprocal interrelating is established which helps create a base on which an effective therapeutic relationship can develop (Truax & Carkhuff, 1967).

Warmth is an elusive quality to define and yet we all know almost immediately when we encounter a "warm" person. Our senses pick up messages of warmth through various aspects of the person, for example, posture (not rigid), facial expression (smiling), gestures (reaching out for a handshake), tone of voice (modulated), eyes (maintains contact), and mood (receptive). As depicted here warmth is experienced for the most part through nonverbal behaviors which tend to stimulate similar responses.

RESPECT

Respect is an elusive concept to define. Egan (1976) believes it means, "prizing another person simply because he is a human being" (p. 147). Respect is more often displayed through behaviors than through words, as rarely do we actually say "I respect you" to a client or a group member. We can, however, convey this message by showing that we value the member's opinions, ideas, hopes, and feelings. Egan further explains the message of respect as an attitude of being "for" the other person. When group members feel others are for them and are treated courteously and considerately as valued persons, they gain a sense of security and feel freer to participate more fully in the group.

FLEXIBILITY

If asked, most people would say they are relatively flexible but if they inquire of someone who knows them well, "Do you think I am flexible?," the person is apt to respond, "Well in some things you are, but in others — well . . . " Pursuing such an interchange can be enlightening and constructive and assists you in evaluating your level and areas of flexibility. By virtue of constantly having to respond to the diverse needs, goals, and limitations of group members a leader-therapist must always be in a state of changeableness. Rarely does the process of a group flow smoothly throughout the session or follow precisely a pre-scribed format. Noncompliance, excitement, dissension, critical incidents, non-attendance, new and absent members can all challenge the plan and the expectations of the session. The leader-therapist must be prepared for these exigencies and be able to respond actively and with flexibility. Other instances where she may need to call on her flexibility could be in:

- Deciding on or changing the task
- Dealing with rules or norms
- Responding to behaviors
- Formalizing structure (i.e., time and place)
- Dealing with other staff
- Coping with peripheral incidents or influences

Collectively the members of a group often form a very diverse assemblage. To be able to interact effectively with so many different personalities requires great flexibility and sensitivity. Diversity may be present in age range as well as in personalities, which can precipitate the need for more flexible rules and limits. Indeed, in many facilities the magnitude of the disparity between adolescents and adults is recognized by the establishment of separate units.

The leader-therapist should keep an open mind to all ideas, alternatives, and methods and try to avoid the we've-always-done-it-this-way manner of thinking. Looking for and responding to new or different ways of "doing" is energizing and stimulates interest and spontaneity.

CREATIVITY AND SPONTANEITY

Closely bound with flexibility is the ability to be creative: to explore new ideas, new methods, and novel approaches. To make the most of such exploring, spontaneity is essential. Just as Moreno believed that spontaneity was crucial to psychodrama, so is it crucial to the group leader. For example, if the group members reach an impasse in a discussion or interchange, try to problem-solve in a creative way. You might think, "Perhaps a role play could be effective"; then act on this idea spontaneously and suggest how the members can get involved. Kottler (1983) notes that "Creative group leaders leave every session bathed in sweat, having squeezed their brains to find new ways of energizing, motivating and facilitating client growth" (p. 94).

To be spontaneous does not mean to be impulsive but rather to have the ability to respond assertively in a variety of ways (Egan, 1976). Assertiveness, but not aggression, is essential to spontaneity. In a postgroup discussion of a particular situation the leader-therapist will sometimes say, "I thought of trying ... but ... " The key is to try it (whatever "it" is), and if it is not effective then feel free to try something else.

ENTHUSIASM

If you are not enthusiastic about the group, then group members are not likely to be enthusiastic either. The result? Probably a very dull, listless, and boring group. As a role model, show interest in the task or discussion, be energetic, get involved, and encourage members to do the same. Enthusiasm means to have a zest and excitement for living, or in this context, for the group experience. Many of your group members, by virtue of their illness or life situations, will have lost their zest, drive, and vitality for life. The enthusiasm you display can be contagious, stirring members to engage in more energetic behaviors and interactions. Leader-therapists are also more likely to get personal satisfaction from the group if they embrace their role enthusiastically rather than if they just go through the motions.

HUMOR

Anything that can be done to lighten the load of fellow sufferers is therapeutic (Tooper, 1984). To be able to laugh at one's own predicaments and help others to see the funny side of theirs is an admirable trait. According to McAdams, Jackson, and Kirshnit (1984), "Looking, laughing, and smiling are powerful nonverbal signals of warmth and attentiveness" (p. 261). Through the use of a good-humored manner leader-therapists can show caring while breaking through the barriers presented by some clients. In the same way, they can model more spontaneous behaviors which clients are then able to imitate. For many clients life has not been a particularly happy experience. Clients with obsessive, schizoid, or depressive characteristics or those who have been ill for a long time especially tend to be grave and solemn (Bloch, Browning & McGrath, 1983).

Even clients with less onerous problems tend to be earnest and anxious. Because of this most group sessions are likely to be serious in tone as members grapple with learning about themselves and their problems. If members can be helped to approach the challenge of changing and learning through a lightening of the mood and by seeing the more humorous aspects of life, then a less arduous process has been facilitated. The relationship between the painful and the humorous can be viewed as paradoxical in that humor can sometimes be used to alleviate the painful (Tooper, 1984). Among the many messages laughter can convey are warmth, insult, friendliness, bitterness, approval, defiance, exuberance, incredulity, nervousness, shame, embarrassment, and ridicule. According to Kottler (1983), laughter is a means of discharge and as an expressed form of communication has much therapeutic value. Group members will sometimes joke and laugh to ease the tension in the group (Orme, 1987) which, depending on the situation, can be either productive or counterproductive. It can be productive if the members are seeking release after an especially intense interchange and the humor serves in a cathartic healing way. Hopefully, there are also times in the group when the members are happy and feeling good and show this by joking, laughing, and just having fun together. However, if the members are joking and laughing to avoid facing up to an intense or important situation, then the process can be counterproductive by allowing the members to ignore the issue at hand.

Egan (1976) qualifies the use of humor as a defense by saying it is "probably the least offensive form of resistance" (p. 154). Joking can not only be used as a way of avoiding the discussion of painful issues, but in some instances can be a means of members bolstering their own self-esteem by putting others down. If this practice is not curtailed it can turn into scapegoating where one member becomes the butt of all the jokes. Such a situation can be very damaging to the member being picked on and requires the prompt intervention of the leader-therapist. Individuals may also use humor as an avoidance technique. One method of doing this is through self-mockery. However, the member that uses self-mockery as a defense mechanism may find other members joining him in his mockery, causing him to feel inadequate and an even stronger need to defend (Bloch, Browning, & McGrath, 1983). Another way that a member may use humor as an avoidance technique is to be the group clown. By constantly joking and clowning around the member is able to keep the other members from taking him or his problems seriously and thus prevents any personal involvement.

At times humor may be introduced through a "fun" task. Banning and Nelson (1987) found that a fun task significantly raised the level of cohesion in groups. In other instances the humorous side of life may only be encountered as the task or discussion unfolds. As long as the leader-therapist does not take herself or her role as leader too seriously, she allows herself and enables others to appreciate the human process with all its foibles.

An opposing view of the use of humor comes as a caution to the leader-therapist against becoming emotionally involved with a member through a humorous exchange which can dull her objective focus on what is being said. This, of course, can happen among members as well as between a member and the leader-therapist. Another problem in using humor, as discussed by Purtilo (1978), is where the leader-therapist and a member use humor as a means of gaining control over each other through a game of one-upmanship. What may start out as seemingly harmless banter can only too easily turn into a sarcastic and punitive interaction. The leader-therapist must always guard against self-aggrandizement at the expense of the members. Therefore, while the presence of humor is usually welcomed by all concerned, its use should be carefully monitored to ensure that a therapeutic process is occurring.

THERAPEUTIC USE OF SELF

Being therapeutic is believed to be more of a personal attribute than a technique and so it is included here. To be therapeutic is really to put all the other attributes into action at the most desirable times to meet the needs and facilitate the achievement of the goals of the members. It is a natural use of the other attributes in a manner that will be helpful rather than harmful.

Another aspect of the therapeutic use of self is the sharing of oneself. This is a controversial issue (Pollak, 1975), and must be engaged in sensitively and thoughtfully. By sharing yourself with the group members you become more of a "person" to them which enables them to more easily identify with you. This identification can lead to members becoming more aware of alternatives, solutions, and coping skills. The caution is to share appropriate information or anecdotes about yourself at appropriate times. If what you share makes you appear too confident or too competent, then you offer an identity that members will believe to be far out of reach for themselves and so they will feel discouraged rather than encouraged. However, these cautious words are not meant to be inhibiting, and every leader-therapist will use herself therapeutically in different ways.

SUMMARY

An effective leader-therapist can be described as being self-confident, responsible, attentive, objective, genuine, empathic, caring, warm, respectful, flexible, creative, enthusiastic, and as having a sense of humor. These personality dimensions as discussed in this chapter are present to a greater or lesser degree in everyone. While some of these attributes can be seen as inherent personality characteristics, such as self-confidence and a sense of humor, most can be learned or enhanced by direct personal efforts. By keeping these characteristics in mind as you analyze your behavior following each group session, you will gain an awareness of your personal strengths and weaknesses and their effect on your functioning as a leader-therapist.

Although "therapeutic use of self" was presented last it is seen to be the most important attribute in becoming an effective leader-therapist. It is also the most difficult attribute to define or describe. It is a way of being that mixes and combines sensitivity, intuition, timing, knowing, and courage with all of the above attributes. This combination represents an active and complex process, but ultimately the degree of success achieved in the role of leader-therapist will depend on how effectively you are able to integrate all facets of yourself into the situation in a therapeutic manner. Having great self-confidence or a keen sense of humor will be irrelevant if you are unable to use these attributes therapeutically in concert with your other attributes and the needs of the situation.

Because of the abstractness of the concept it is difficult to delineate what must be learned in order to achieve what is termed the therapeutic use of self. However, from the awareness gained through ongoing self-analysis and self-exploration you can direct your efforts for personal change toward increasing, improving, and integrating your areas of competency while decreasing any inhibiting attributes. Through this gradual process of change there is likely to evolve a leader-therapist who continues to enhance her therapeutic use of self.

CHAPTER 7

Leadership Techniques

> *Verbal communication is usually a lie. The real communication is beyond words.*
>
> — FRITZ PERLS

The attributes discussed in Chapter 6 are primarily personal characteristics, whereas techniques and strategies are more methods of leadership and constitute skills that can be learned. This is not to say that the leader-therapist should have a bag of tricks from which she pulls out interventions in a hit-or-miss fashion. Indeed, Corey (1982) cautions, "It is impossible to overemphasize that techniques cannot be effectively used if they are things that are grabbed onto" (p. 241). The leader-therapist must become knowledgeable about certain techniques and how they can facilitate both group and individual progress. She will then use these techniques selectively and appropriately in promoting therapeutic outcomes. For any leader-therapist the most effective techniques will be those that are congruent with her own personal style of leadership and are an extension of her natural "therapeutic use of self." Such effective leadership involves a combination of affective, cognitive, and behavioral techniques (Corey, 1982). The leader must be sensitive to and able to perceive each group member individually as well as the group as a whole. She must comprehend what is happening and then, when appropriate or necessary, be facilitative by employing the most appropriate technique.

The "what is happening" is called the process, and following this on an ongoing basis is called processing. Loomis (1979) says, "Group therapists . . . have described the process of their groups in terms of insight, interpersonal learning, catharsis and corrective emotional experience" (p. 27). Thus the leader, while being *a part* of the group, must always also be *apart* from the group, constantly observing the process. As discussed earlier in this text, process involves to whom and in what manner members say things, nonverbal behaviors such as facial expressions and body movements, voice tones and inflections, and reactions and feelings. However, it is not enough to only perceive what is occurring in the group; the leader must also help the members to acquire some cognitive understanding of the process in order for them to benefit from the experience. Yalom (1983) calls this the "illumination of process," and believes it must coexist with the here-and-now interactions for the group to be therapeutic. In order to help members understand the process, and to affect and promote the process, there are techniques and strategies that a leader-therapist should be skilled in.

RESTATEMENT

To restate what a member has said is basically to repeat his communication using similar language and syntax. The purpose of using this technique is to convey to the member that you are paying close attention and have heard what he has said (Trotzer, 1977). It also serves to encourage the member to expand or say more. Example:

Statement: I wish I had more energy as my wife is getting fed up with me.

Restatement: You wish you felt more energetic as your wife is feeling fed up with you.

Following the restatement the member may go on to explain the effects of his low energy level on other aspects of his life, to describe his wife's "fed up" behaviors, or expand on his overall problems.

A situation where restating can be particularly useful is if a member is speaking and becomes distracted. When you restate what he just said it prods him to continue speaking. It is not a difficult skill to learn but can become sterile and boring if overused.

REFLECTION

Reflecting is the ability to convey the meaning of a member's contribution in such a way as to demonstrate that you both heard and understood. Reflections are not as superficial as restatements. They can focus on the content of what was said or they can reflect the feelings that underlay the communication. Another factor contributing to the complexity of this skill is that it encompasses both verbal and nonverbal messages. Reflecting nonverbal communications can be surprising and enlightening to a member and needs to be done with sensitivity as, used in this way, reflecting can be threatening (Trotzer, 1977). For example, if a member is trying to hide behind a stream of bright chatter but the sadness he really feels is displayed in his facial expression and the latter is reflected by the leader-therapist then the person can feel "found out" and vulnerable. Reflections of lesser impact could be the following:

Statement: I just want to get out of here and go back to work.

Reflection: It sounds like you have had enough of this place and would like to get on with your life.

Observation: *Member is shifting in his chair, crossing and uncrossing his legs, swinging his feet.*

Reflection: It seems like you can't get comfortable as you are fidgeting a lot today.

In reflecting feelings the leader must not appear to be *telling* a member what he is feeling but rather to be *checking* on what the member is feeling. If a member says, "You don't care about me. If you did you would remember my wife's name," and you respond with, "You feel that if I remembered your wife's name you would know that I cared about you," then you leave the communication line open for the member to continue and say more about what he is feeling. If you respond to the above with, "That's not true. Of course I care about you. It's just that I'm very poor at remembering names," then you tend to end the communication and the member is less likely to continue. Or on observing that Mary's eyes are watering and she has stopped talking the leader might say, "Mary, you look upset." This reflection allows Mary to (a) agree that she is upset (which may lead to a discussion of why she is upset) or (b) deny she is upset (which could lead to exploring just what Mary is feeling).

Occasionally a leader-therapist can be facilitative by reflecting on the behavior of the group overall, as follows:

Leader-therapist: It seems like everyone is talking at once!

This is an especially useful technique to use if the group members become so caught up in content that they are oblivious of the process. Reflection at this point not only causes a pause in the action of the group but can also be facilitative in producing change.

As with the use of restatement, caution is required to prevent the overuse of reflection which, when carried to its extreme, can become what Corey and Corey (1982) refer to as a "hollow echo." These authors believe that reflection may be a good beginning technique but should be followed by more exploratory interventions. In the following example the first response is a straight reflection, whereas the second includes speculation about causative factors.

Statement: I have to set a date for our wedding pretty soon as Sue won't wait forever.

Reflective response: It sounds like you are afraid Sue might change her mind if you don't agree on a wedding date soon.

Exploratory response: It sounds like you are afraid Sue might change her mind but you are still not sure you want to get married.

The exploratory response can be slightly personal and challenging and is more likely to precipitate further dialogue than is the straight reflective response.

PARAPHRASING

Paraphrasing is similar to reflection, which not only makes it easy to confuse the two but hampers differentiating between them clearly. Paraphrasing addresses the major communication problem that occurs when people assume that what they understood another person to say is actually what the other person intended to say. In responding to others most people speak from their own understanding of what the other person meant without checking to see if they *heard* the message or the intention correctly. On hearing a new telephone number, we often repeat it to check for accuracy, but with other communications we usually assume that we heard correctly what was said.

In order to make sure that the meaning you take from another person's remark is the meaning that he intended, you can check by asking, "Can you clarify that?," or, "Is this [statement] what you meant?" You can also paraphrase what was said to show the other person what his statement meant to you, for example:

Member: My husband is very nasty to me.

Leader-therapist: He physically abuses you?

Member: No, he doesn't do that, but he constantly laughs and sneers at me.

The above paraphrase by the leader leads to a clarification of what the member ment by "nasty." However, if the leader had said, "He is mean to you?," the member might have said "Yes," but the leader would still not know specifically what the husband does when he is being nasty and may assume that he physically abuses the member. So when paraphrasing it is very important to be specific, to try to define exactly what the other person is saying.

Another reason that paraphrasing is a useful tool in communication is that it conveys interest in the other person. It is evidence that you want to understand what the other person is saying. Because paraphrasing does convey a message of interest the other person may be more inclined to open up and share. Paraphrasing comes from a genuine desire to understand what another person means and is one of the best ways to increase accuracy in communication.

CLARIFYING

The responsibility of clarifying what an individual member says or what the group is doing often falls to the leader. You can be sure that if you do not understand something that has been said or done there will be others who do not understand. They, however, may not feel comfortable saying so. In such instances it is important to facilitate understanding by clarifying. When Joe says, "I don't want to be in group," it is not clear whether he is uncomfortable with this particular session, has something pressing he wants to do right now, or he just generally dislikes being part of the group. If let pass, such an ambiguous statement by Joe can affect how the other members relate to him. To clarify you might ask, "Joe, do you mean just today?". Hopefully, his answer will clear up the confusion surrounding his previous statement, enabling everyone to feel more comfortable with Joe and the situation.

Sometimes clarifying the overall process in the group is required. If the members seem to be going in different directions with the discussion or task, the question, "Can someone explain what we are doing right now?," may precipitate clarification and render a clearer focus. Other clarifiers might be, "Is the problem deciding who will do what?," or, "Have we decided on how to begin?" Intervening in these or similar ways can be facilitative in helping members define immediate goals and decide how to proceed. There are times when members will get caught up in a game of semantics and then a clarifying statement can often end the confusion. Sampson and Marthas (1981) see the role of the leader "as being primarily to introduce questions that cause members to focus on their own process of interaction" (p. 233). Paraphrasing, as discussed previously, can also be an effective method of clarifying.

SUPPORT

Offering support is a means of encouraging an individual member or the group as a whole. Support should be proffered in both good times and bad times, that is, when the group (or a member) is thought to be doing well, and when they (or a member) appear to be in difficulty. There will be times when a person, finding it painful to explore an issue or deal with a situation, appears to stop or pull back. This could be an instance where offering some support is appropriate and appreciated. To be supportive the leader-therapist might say something like, "It's difficult to deal with such a tough issue by yourself. Maybe we can help." To the group, the leader might offer encouragement (e.g., "As a group you are working very hard and I'm sure it's not easy"). Supportive statements let the group (member) know that: (a) you are listening; (b) what they are saying is valued; (c) you are aware of their feelings.

Sometimes this is all that is necessary for the group or member to feel able to carry on. Feeling confident that what they say will be recognized and responded to they feel more comfortable in continuing or initiating. Creating a supportive climate in the group is important in enabling the members to feel comfortable in sharing their ideas and feelings and in exploring new avenues. It is more likely that members will share what they deem to be the unacceptable parts of themselves or their lives in a supportive environment. By offering supportive comments at appropriate times, the leader-therapist serves as a role model, and group members may then follow suit by being supportive of their peers. However, giving support at inappropriate times, such as when a member is looking for unwarranted sympathy or is being overly dependent, can be counterproductive. The skill then is not only in being able to be supportive but in knowing when such an intervention will be therapeutic.

TIMING

We have all heard it said that a certain person's "timing was right" and that is why he was successful or why things went so well for him. Similarly, in a group, for things to go well, the timing of interventions is a crucial factor. Although timing is one of the most important skills for a leader-therapist to develop (Hansen, Warner, & Smith, 1976), there are no rules to follow or guidelines to go by. Skill in this technique comes with practice and experience. The following points may serve as useful guidelines.

As with all leadership techniques, timing must be based on the process occurring in the group at the time. Any intervention must be congruent with what is going on in the group at that particular moment. More specifically, the intervention must be congruent with the personal state of any specific individual who is directly involved (Mahler, 1969). For example, if a member is still very defensive and the leader-therapist pushes a point, the intervention may only serve to make the member more defensive. So, not only must the intervention be congruent but it should be made at the *optimal* time. To intervene too early in a discussion can cut off or stifle the interaction, but to wait too long is to risk losing the facilitative aspect of the intervention. For instance, if feelings are building among members in the group and the leader intervenes too early, then the members can opt out by entering into interaction with the leader rather than continuing the discussion with one another. This allows their feelings to dissipate and resolution can be lost. However, at other times it will be more productive for the leader to make the intervention early in order to prevent feelings from escalating. The skill is to recognize the differences in the two situations and to intervene accordingly.

In considering another kind of group where the discussion is more one of brainstorming or idea exchange, the leader faces the same question of when (if at all) to intervene. In this case you might look for more objective criteria: (a) Are group members getting too far off the topic? (b) Is the interaction among the members more important (for the moment) than staying on the topic? and (c) Are most members or only a few involved in the exchange? Weighing these or other factors will help the leader decide when and how to intervene. Often you will be able to tell from the reaction of the group members whether your timing was facilitative or not. If members ignore your input you can pretty well conclude that your timing was off. Conversely, if the group responds by incorporating your input and carrying on, then you have probably been on target.

It is said elsewhere in this book, but is worthy of repeating, that as a rule of thumb it is better to err on the side of too few interventions than too many. New leaders often tend to be too active because they feel responsible for keeping the group going and attempt to do so by intervening or contributing in some manner. A situation that tends to precipitate poorly timed interventions by a novice leader-therapist is when there is protracted silence in the group. Because of the degree of their discomfort, new leaders frequently have a distorted sense of the duration of the silence and believe it to be much longer than it is in fact.

A last important point about timing is the *time* itself. The leader needs to keep an eye on the clock to ensure sufficient time is left to allow for a smooth approach to closure. If the members are into a heavy discussion and group time is almost up, it is important to intervene in an effort to help members resolve the issue and deal with their individual feelings within the remaining time. In some facilities, due to staff or program requirements, groups must stop exactly on time. If members are left feeling up in the air because of unfinished business, this can be unproductive, both for them individually and for the milieu of the group. Sometimes, but again not always, it is helpful to let the group know how much time is remaining and to indicate the need to finish up ("There is 5 minutes left so we need to think about closing," or "We have 10 minutes left to share our thoughts and feelings on this"). The value of such interventions depends on what is going on in the group at the time and the manner in which a particular intervention is made. In certain instances such an intervention can inhibit members' participation and the group may come to an abrupt end. At other times it may facilitate members to get to the point, make decisions, or move to supportive and summary comments bringing the group to a comfortable and productive close.

PROBING AND QUESTIONING

Many of the personal qualities and therapeutic skills that produce a successful interview are the same as those required to effect a productive group session. Because of this similarity and because therapists are used to interviewing it is very easy for the leader-therapist to fall into an interview format with individual members of the group. For the leader-therapist to become involved at great length in such a didactic interaction is detrimental to group process as it tends to exclude the other group members. The techniques of probing and questioning are the ones most likely to draw a leader-therapist into an interviewlike situation with a group member.

Aside from the risks just mentioned, probing can enable group members to explore and expand their awareness in order to reach deeper levels of understanding. It is useful in encouraging members to generate new ideas and alternatives, to aid in developing the topic, and to promote deeper levels of relating. Probing can take the form of direct questions, statements, or phrases.

- How did that make you feel?
- That sounds stressful.
- And then?

As with the other techniques, the leader-therapist must use probing with a good deal of sensitivity. It can be very threatening to group members and if done too directly or forcefully members can feel pushed or picked on, and they may withdraw or respond defensively.

STATEMENTS VERSUS QUESTIONS

In carrying out your role of leader-therapist, posing questions to group members is inevitable and can be productive. Three types of questions are defined by Potter and Anderson (1970): (1) closed-end; (2) directive; and (3) open-end. The question, "How would the group like to handle it?," is open-end and more facilitative than, "Would you like to go around the circle taking turns?," which is a closed-end question. You may get a variety of responses and ideas to the first question, but probably only a yes or no from the second question. The second question keeps you in the position of control whereas the first gives control to the group and lets them decide what to do. A directive question requests information about ideas being discussed, for example, "What are the advantages of the group meeting in the afternoon?" Directive questions are useful in encouraging members to explore alternatives and assess the options.

Every question has two aspects, cognitive and affective (Potter & Anderson, 1970). A respondent's answer will be determined by his assessment of and reaction to these two aspects. If the attitude of the questioner is blaming or hostile ("Why are you late for group this time?"), it could well elicit a defensive answer. A softer, gently enquiring question ("Did something happen this morning that made you late for group?") may engender more open and honest information. Since the affective aspects have much to do with voice tone and facial expression the differences in the questions are difficult to depict here with only the written word.

Statements can also be productive. The statement, "I think we could explore this further," is more likely to produce further discussion than, "Do you think we have covered the issue?" The latter has more of a closing-off tone, whereas the first denotes a sense of opening up. This is not to say there are not times when you do want to close off the discussion and therefore would deliberately choose to use the question rather than the statement.

The directing as well as the phrasing of questions has important implications. Asking questions of a specific member of the group may invite a one-to-one interaction with the member. Of course this cannot always be avoided nor need it be. There are times when issues need to be explored with certain members or specific individuals need to be drawn out. Points to ponder at these times are the duration of the dialogue, whether the rest of the group is excluded, and if the content of the discussion can be broadened to include some of the other members. Variety, considered to be the spice of life, can also be considered as the spice of questions and statements. Shoemaker's (1987) research demonstrates that by "varying the focus of interventions and the pattern of communication" (p. 36), the leader-therapist can significantly affect the type of learning that occurs. Keeping inquiries varied and fresh will contribute to input and interaction being more stimulating and provocative.

CONTENT VERSUS PROCESS

As mentioned previously it is crucial that you be constantly aware of the dynamics unfolding in the group. Included should be an awareness of how you are affecting the group and how you are being affected by the group. Concurrent to being *aware* of the process you must *monitor* the process, be it a discussion or an active task. Sometimes, a member will bring up an issue or topic having great relevance and interest to you personally. In such instances there can be a natural tendency to get completely caught up in the discussion, to forget your leadership role as you become totally involved with the content. This can present a problem in that it leaves no one to mind the store and as *you* become more active other group members may pull back. At this point you may find yourself in the position of "lecturing" to the group on your favorite topic, or sliding into an exclusive one-to-one discussion with a particular member. So, while it is important to pay attention and be involved in the content, it is equally important to remain observant and objective.

BITING YOUR TONGUE

I think it can safely be said that for the most part occupational therapists are a gregarious lot. They use their friendliness to great advantage in motivating patients to work and comply with treatment goals. It can also be useful in groups to create a comfortable and friendly atmosphere. However, this very trait can make it difficult as leader-therapist to watch your group flounder and not jump in to bail them out. Difficult as it may be, biting your tongue is often the most productive course to take. It is stressful to do this because as therapists we are used to solving problems, directing treatment, and generally participating actively with our clients. On average, in a group setting, it is usually more productive for your members, both individually and as a group, to work things out and solve their own problems. It may take them longer, doing it themselves, but their gains in learning and the added feelings of competency are very rewarding.

FEEDBACK

People seek feedback because it is a way of evaluating their attitudes, behaviors, ideas, feelings, and physical attributes. It is the means by which people can "learn about and 'validate' themselves" (Snyder, Ingram, Handelsman, & Wells, 1982, p. 317). According to Samovar and Mills (1976) the term *feedback* refers to reactions obtained from your listeners and the efforts you make in adapting to these perceived reactions. One simple example of this process is when a group member is told, "I can't hear you," and the member receiving this message responds by speaking louder. Although it is generally assumed that most people welcome feedback it should be kept in mind that people do differ in the *degree* of their desire for feedback. This means that some group members will be more receptive to receiving feedback than will others and it is important, as leader, to be prepared for varied reactions. People also tend to accept positive feedback and believe in its accuracy more readily than they do negative feedback (Handelsman & Snyder, 1982), and therefore the latter is more likely to precipitate defensive behavior.

The well-known lines of Robert Burns, "O wad some power the giftie gie us, to see oursel's as ithers see us," intimate our hunger to know how others perceive us. People want to know how they are seen by others in order to validate or, at times, invalidate their self-perceptions. Group members have the opportunity to meet these needs when a feedback process is activated in the group. They can determine the effects of their behaviors and ways of interrelating with others from the feedback they receive. Having more than his own point of view can be seen as advantageous in the cognitive structuring or restructuring of a person's behavior. In emphasizing the importance of the feedback process Bernard (1974) says, "Feedback may be negative, positive or equivocal but it is essential to normal functioning" (p. 289). Giving feedback is a skill (Egan, 1976) requiring sensitivity. By keeping the following points in mind you will facilitate a more meaningful and effective feedback process.

1. Be sensitive to what information the group is ready to use. Give feedback that will be most helpful *to the group* at the time. The behaviors and incidents observed as most significant by *you* will not necessarily be the ones the group is ready to hear about.

2. Do not "avalanche" the group with information. If too much information is given at one time the group will find it overwhelming and barely useful. Because of their confusion the members may even ignore all the feedback.

3. Do not overpraise the group. Be selective and give praise on specifics; otherwise members may feel they have "made it" and therefore need make no further efforts.

4. Try not to punish, preach, or judge. Instead of saying, "Some of you dominated the discussion today," say, "It was interesting that participation was less general today than it was last session."

5. Feedback should be immediate. Give feedback when the behavior occurs rather than waiting until the end of the group to comment. Saying, "That was a very helpful suggestion Mary," "I find it very distracting when you keep tapping your fingers," or, "You are very quiet to-day," allows the member in question an opportunity to repeat or change his behavior during the remainder of the group.

6. Use confrontive feedback carefully in the beginning of a group. Early confrontation can frighten members and inhibit them from further participation. This is not to say that disruptive behaviors should be overlooked during this time. They should be confronted immediately or as warranted.

7. Act as a role model for giving feedback:

> **Leader:** [*To John*] I'm finding it difficult to concentrate when you keep tapping your fingers. [*To group*] "Is it bothering anyone else?
>
> **Member:** Yes
>
> **Leader:** Could you tell John that?

By speaking to John yourself initially you demonstrate that it is acceptable to give this sort of feedback and members will then feel more comfortable in following your lead.

Feedback can be given to the group as a whole as well as to individuals. It helps to keep the group focused (e.g., "We seem to be getting off topic"), balances affect with content ("You seem to be avoiding saying how you feel about these issues"), and clarifies process ("I notice that John always speaks for the group"). In all cases feedback should be descriptive rather than evaluative or judgmental. In addition, it is most useful when it has a here-and-now rather than a there-and-then focus (Blumberg & Golembiewski, 1976). It is more difficult to deny or argue with behaviors that can be pinpointed and described as they occur. Once their existence has been established, then their effect on then-and-there situations can be hypothesized and discussed.

CONFRONTATION

Confrontation is also a form of feedback. Whether a member says a benign, "You are speaking too softly," or a much stronger, "You interrupted me," the member is functioning in a confrontational role. Confrontation is a means of prompting individuals to examine their behaviors, of breaking through defenses, and of increasing awareness. It is a skill requiring practice to ensure that its use will be facilitative and not destructive. Unfortunately, the word confrontation has a rather negative connotation, but the actual act of confronting need not produce a negative experience for those involved. In confronting a member or the group you can be straightforward and direct, but you need not be abrasive. One of the main things to be aware of in confronting another person is your tone of voice. An even, low voice will help to present your confrontation in a sensitive and caring way. Four components of constructive confrontation offered by Kreps and Thornton (1984) are: (1) clarifying the issue, (2) expressing feelings descriptively, (3) expressing facts and fantasies, and (4) resolution and agreement (p. 186). These are in keeping with the previous suggestions for offering constructive feedback.

The leader-therapist can use confrontation as a means of letting an individual or the whole group know that she is aware of what is going on. In this way she can make her point while simultaneously serving as a role model in demonstrating confrontive behaviors for the group members. For example, in a certain group a member called Tony is always blaming others or poor circumstances for his problems and what he sees as his misfortunes. The leader-therapist believes that the other members are aware of Tony's behavior but are reluctant to confront him. The following illustrates how she might deal with the situation:

Tony: I didn't get the job because the fellow who interviewed me didn't ask the right questions and he ended the interview too soon.

Leader-therapist: Tony, I feel we've heard this from you before. When things go wrong for you it always seems to be someone else's fault.

Tony: Well it was. If he'd asked me the right questions and given me more time I could have got the job.

Leader-therapist: Tony, you are still blaming someone else and this seems to be the way that you often react to avoid accepting responsibility for your own behavior. Let's hear what the others think about what you've said.

With the leader-therapist's second response she is making an interpretation of Tony's behavior as a means of emphasizing the point to be made. In doing this she may initiate an involved one-to-one interaction with Tony which could exclude the rest of the group. By referring the issue to the group, as she does at the end of her second response, she will hopefully extricate herself from the dialogue while stimulating the group members to follow on with their feedback to Tony. This can strengthen the message to be conveyed.

Most importantly, any confrontation should "manifest your concern for the other" (Egan, 1983). Used punitively or insensitively, it is sure to cause the individual or the group to retreat. Confrontation should always convey caring and function as a means of increasing involvement.

ANALYSIS AND INTERPRETATION

Observation is the forerunner to analysis, and analysis is the forerunner to interpretation. It is important to separate observations from interpretations. The leader-therapist must be able to separate what she sees and hears from what she thinks these observations mean (Sampson & Marthas, 1981). She should not be hasty in making interpretations but should analyze her observations over time and under the circumstances. For example, if John is smiling you might infer that he is happy, but on further observation you find that John also smiles when he is being confronted or is relating a sad experience. On analyzing several of these situations you might then conclude that John uses smiling as a defense mechanism. Interpreted, this could mean that John is unable or unwilling to experience or express his real feelings. Continued interaction with John may supply more clues and information on which to base further interpretations.

It is important to present any interpretation as a hunch or a hypothesis rather than a statement of fact. Therefore interpretations are often prefaced with the words "it seems" or "it appears." This way the validity of the interpretation is open to agreement or disagreement, acceptance or rejection by the member involved. An interpretation, if accurate, can be useful in moving a member or the group past an impasse as it opens up a new way of looking at or evaluating the situation or issue (Corey & Corey, 1982). Interpretation is frequently used to help persons gain insight into why they behave the way they do. It is most often used in the psychoanalytic approach to psychotherapy, but is a useful technique for any leader-therapist. To make an inaccurate interpretation is not a calamity. The member or group will usually set you straight about your error and then together you can explore other possibilities. Even when your interpretation is judged to be off base, there is the possibility that it contains a grain of truth which could give the member or group some food for thought. The leader-therapist need not always be the one to make an interpretation. In some cases it may be more beneficial for the member to attempt to interpret his own behavior. The leader-therapist might encourage the member to do so by saying,

"John, what do you think is the reason that you always make a joke when Bill talks about his mother?"

In analyzing what is going on in the group or with individuals, many aspects must be considered: the order and context of events, interrelationships, nonverbal behaviors, verbal behaviors, actions, and affect. Good observational skills, steady concentration, and acute awareness are all necessary in order to absorb and analyze the total dynamics of the group. Sometimes presenting the analysis to the group will motivate the members themselves to examine what is going on in the group. For example, a group is trying to decide what its task will be for the next session, but each time they get close to making a decision they begin to vacillate and then pull back. By making this observation you are presenting the group with an analysis of what you perceive to be happening in the group. You are not saying *why* it is happening, but only that it *is* happening. Such an analysis can be effective in breaking up the pattern of behaviors occurring in the group and moving the members on to more productive behaviors. Group analysis is discussed more fully in Chapter 10.

SUMMARIZING

Although we usually associate a summary with completion, it can be useful to summarize at various points during a group. If the group has exhausted a topic or is floundering, summarizing what has been discussed can help the members decide if there is more to be said or if it is time to move on (Trotzer, 1977). To summarize the points made by various group members can be especially facilitative if the group is involved in a decision making process or in a task requiring several steps. The summary can prod the group to complete one step or begin the next one.

Near the close of a session you might make a summary statement about how you thought the group went, and check if your perceptions match those of the members. Another way of summarizing is to discuss how you are feeling at the close of the session and invite others to do the same. This helps to assess how members are feeling before they leave the group as a check for unfinished business or unresolved feelings.

SUMMARY

A leader-therapist will be most effective if she can remain objective and guard against getting personally caught up in either the content or the process. She can do this by monitoring both areas separately and continually, and then when appropriate, respond to the needs of each with facilitative techniques. This is not to say that she should not offer herself personally or that she should refrain from contributing. However, it does mean that entering into an argument with a member or telling the group what the right answer or right way is can, in the former instance, be a destructive maneuver, and in the latter, be inhibiting to the sharing of ideas. Becoming personally involved also takes the leader-therapist out of the role of observer and places her in the role of *powerful member* — powerful because of her given role of leader-therapist. This latter role carries great influence as well as the concept of knowing, and therefore she is often perceived by members to be an "expert." Usually it is more productive to observe and facilitate the process among members than to intervene as an expert and risk terminating it. Members may take time to get it right, but they are more likely to retain any learning that occurs if they go through the process themselves.

In addition to the personal characteristics (discussed in Chapter 6) that are conducive to effective leadership, there are techniques and strategies that can be learned and used as ongoing methods or at appropriate junctures during a group session. The techniques presented here facilitate interaction processes and outcomes. Some, such as supporting, clarifying, questioning, and biting your tongue, will be more familiar and hence more comfortable to use than others. As a rule, normal, accepted social skills do not include confronting, probing, giving feedback, or analyzing or interpreting the behavior of others and so these techniques, besides requiring theoretical knowledge, may require conscious practice. Still other techniques, specifically restatement, reflection, and paraphrasing, contribute to more effective communication and increased understanding between participators, and skill with the use of these techniques can enhance any relationship.

CHAPTER 8

What to Do If . . .

> *You cannot create experience,*
> *you must undergo it.*
> — ALBERT CAMUS

Each group session is unique. Even with the same members no two sessions will ever present the same dynamics nor can one predict how the process will evolve. You may speculate on behaviors of certain members, but because the process is constantly changing, individual members frequently react differently given new situations. Therefore, as leader-therapist you must always be prepared for the unexpected. Unusual and unique events must be dealt with as they arise. There are, however, some situations and incidents that occur often enough to be considered common occurrences. By thinking and planning ahead you will be better prepared to deal with them when the time comes.

MEMBER-TO-LEADER-THERAPIST DIALOGUE

In any situation where a leader is involved, the members of the group tend to look to that leader for guidance. Members will wait for the leader to give direction. In small therapy groups an effective leader-therapist tries to relinquish this directive role as quickly as possible. She tries to get the members to involve themselves with one another and to assume responsibility for the decision making and overall functioning of the group. In therapeutic groups members not only look to the leader-therapist for direction but also for help with their personal issues. This is understandable since the clients perceive the group as a treatment measure and staff as the persons who are the most knowledgeable, most understanding, and most able to respond or help. Other reasons for which members turn exclusively to the leader-therapist are to impress the staff member with their good behavior or their efforts to participate, to try to establish an individual relationship with the leader-therapist, or because of their uncertainty about the reactions, responses, and acceptance of the other members. However, for the leader-therapist to enter into one-to-one dialogues with different members defeats the whole concept and purpose of the group as a therapeutic modality.

Members tend to turn to the leader-therapist more frequently at the beginning of a session when the group is functioning in the dependency stage. Later on in the session, instances that may precipitate a one-to-one interchange developing are when the leader-therapist enters the discussion to clarify, comment, or ask a question. This brings the focus of the group or of a particular member back to the leader-therapist, creating potential for a limiting dialogue to develop.

Dialogues such as these are seen as hazardous because they usually exclude the other group members and hence there is a risk of losing them. The other members may lose interest in what is going on, as it does not involve them directly, and they may respond by tuning out. Another possible reaction, especially if your one-to-one interaction is lengthy, is that other members may begin to whisper and interact among themselves. When this occurs you face the problem of re-engaging the members, yourself, and the individual member you were talking with into a unified whole again. If this happens several times during a session, the group unity or "we-ness" becomes fragmented, resulting in the growth and development of the group as a unit being retarded.

Unfortunately, it is all too easy to fall into a one-to-one interaction as the therapist in us wants out and wants to help the client. Feeding into this need as well is the desire of the member to receive what he sees as expert help. As previously mentioned, members usually see the leader-therapist as more *knowing* than the other group members and therefore what she has to say is perceived to be more valuable. Now it could be argued that what the leader has to say might be more valuable and pertinent than what a member might say, but this is not the point. The point is to involve the group members with one another, to trust in the group process for the benefit of all. The members may not be as perceptive, insightful, or articulate as the leader-therapist, but together they have the potential for dealing with an individual member or a problem quite productively (Shapiro, 1978). Members helping and being helped is a two-way process that brings out altruistic tendencies. By observing and being involved in the problem solving of others, members can gain insight into their own problems and behaviors (Trotzer, 1977).

There are several things the leader-therapist can do to avoid getting caught up in a lengthy one-to-one interaction or to extricate herself once she has become involved. The best preventive measure is to try always to be aware of the overall group process, including her own manner of interacting. The importance of the unwritten rule, "think process," cannot be overemphasized. The following are other measures, both preventive and active, that can be employed.

BREAKING EYE CONTACT

Most people prefer to talk to someone who maintains eye contact with them (Barker, 1981). This fact can have relevance when you find yourself caught up in a one-to-one interaction that you feel is not productive for the group as a whole. You can try casually glancing away from the member and he, having lost eye contact with you, will most likely look around the group in hopes of establishing eye contact with someone else. This glancing away can be achieved without rudeness or conveying rejection and the chances are another member will respond, which sets up a member-member interaction. When this happens there is an increased possibility of other members joining in. Group members are more likely to enter into an ongoing conversation between two members than they are to enter into an interaction between the leader-therapist and a member. In the latter instance members may feel that they are interrupting or interfering with therapy if they attempt to get involved.

REDIRECTING

Sometimes you can terminate a one-to-one interaction by redirecting the member to the group. If the member is questioning you or seeking advice, then you can say, as you gesture around the group, "What do others think?," or, "John, how about asking the other members about that?," or, "I'm sure the other members could help you with that." This same technique can also be successful if the member is telling you about a specific issue of his. You can suggest that he share his problem with the group (e.g., "I'm sure someone here has had a similar problem or experience"), and then look to the group for response. In this way you encourage members to interact more with one another and enhance the value of what they have to say. You can always make your point or give your response later if you think it is important and has not already been mentioned.

Members frequently talk to the leader *about* other group members ("I think Mary is . . ."). This usually happens because members are afraid that what they have to say may upset their fellow group member. By channeling their input through the leader-therapist they feel somewhat protected. Members are more apt to talk about another member rather than to the other member at the beginning of a group because the ground rules have not yet been established. If such an instance arises you can direct the member who is talking to you about Mary to speak directly *to* Mary with, "John, I think it's important for you to tell that *to* Mary." Initially members will feel a bit awkward or embarrassed by your request, but they usually comply and quickly learn this more direct and productive way of interacting.

LAST-MINUTE INPUT

Not infrequently you will have a member bring up an important issue just before the group is scheduled to end. This may be due to several factors: the member finds it difficult to speak out but on realizing that the session is almost over he finds the courage to blurt out his problem; the member vacillates throughout the group trying to decide if he should mention his problem and then with time running out he finally decides to do so; the member takes a long time in formalizing what he wants to say; or the member's issue is not compatible with the day's topic and that is why he has not had an opportunity to bring it up earlier. Whatever the reason, the leader-therapist is left to deal with a member sharing something very important to him with little, if any, time left. Depending on the issue and the urgency you might (a) tell the member that the group will discuss the issue at the beginning of the next group, (b) try to respond quickly and as best you can in the time remaining, (c) suggest that the member talk to one of the ward staff about the issue, or (d) ask if there is a member who would talk with the individual after group and have both report this discussion back to the group at the next session. If your schedule permits and you think the problem is urgent you could discuss it with the member after group. This solution, however, can engender future problems when members realize the benefits of bringing issues up at the close of a session. The benefit, of course, is the leader-therapist's undivided attention in a one-to-one dialogue after group.

THE MONOPOLIST

You will probably expend more energy as a leader trying to get members to talk and participate than vice versa, but occasionally you will have an overtalkative member. Such a person can be a problem for two reasons. First, the overtalkative member uses up so much air time that other members may give up trying to participate. Second, quiet members may find the overparticipator to be a blessing in disguise. His domination lets them off the hook, allowing them to remain quiet and remote. There are several techniques that may be successful in attempting to equalize air time among members.

RECOGNITION AND "GATEKEEPING"

You can recognize a member's contribution by giving positive feedback to the member, as with, "Mary, you have given us some very good ideas. Now let's hear what the others have to say." As you say the latter sentence you physically turn to the other members, inviting them to contribute. Figuratively speaking, this opens the gate to let them in. This technique, known as "gatekeeping," can be quite effective. While the talkative member takes a minute to bask in your praise, hopefully another (or several) member(s) will respond.

TAKING TURNS

If you are aware of the talkative member (from previous groups) you can select an activity for the session that requires going around the circle and having each member give his or her contribution in turn. This way you have some control over the air time, as you can then say, "Sorry Mary, but we are going around the group and it's now Jim's turn." Even if you do not have a task that requires taking turns, you can institute such a process in a free discussion by saying, "Let's go around the circle with each of you giving your thoughts and feelings so we'll be sure to hear from everyone."

NONVERBAL CONTACT

Again, if you are aware of the member's monopolizing behavior before group begins, you can arrange to sit beside him. If there is no vacant seat beside him it is perfectly all right to suggest a change of seats during group. Be sure to explain why you are making the switch. A comment such as, "John, you are pretty active in group so I think it might be helpful if I sit beside you," is all that is required. The close proximity of sitting beside a group member gives you an excellent opportunity to exert unobtrusive monitoring of the monopolist's behavior. It allows you to nonverbally help the member regulate his input. A slight touch on the arm or hand can be sufficient to deter the monopolist from interrupting or speaking at inappropriate times. A finger to your lips as you turn to the member can gently give him the message that he should be quiet. This method of control is more likely to give the member the feeling that you are *with* him rather than *against* him or *getting at* him. It is a means of conveying caring, while eliminating the need to speak to him across the group, which is likely to focus the whole group's attention on him. This method of being beside and with a member will be mentioned again in the section on dealing with a psychotic patient.

CONFRONTATION

When you have tried the aforementioned techniques without success, or if the monopolist's behavior is very disruptive and you feel immediate action is required, you might want to use a more confrontive approach: "John, I'm wondering if you are aware of how much you have been talking in group this morning. We appreciate your ideas but it is important that others also have a chance to speak." If John relapses into monopolizing later in the group you can again point out his disruptive behavior and offer to help him in controlling it: "John, you still seem to be having trouble controlling your talking so I'm going to sit beside you to help you remember to let others have their say." Then move to sit beside John and use the nonverbal techniques mentioned above. With human nature being so varied, some clients will not be as responsive to your requests or suggestions as others. For unresponsive members you may elect to set more limits and be more confrontive, in order to prevent them from totally disrupting the group. It is best to be direct and firm, but even-toned and sensitive, in your statements.

THE NONPARTICIPATOR

There are many reasons why a member may be quiet in group but the most common one is that the member is feeling too intimidated to speak out. Other reasons can be that he has nothing to say that is pertinent to the discussion, that he is upset about a personal matter and does not feel like participating at that particular time, or that he feels inadequate and therefore feels he has nothing worthwhile to say. Still others refrain from speaking out of fear of exposing themselves, or because they feel they can maintain their distance from the group through silence. In some cases the member may remain silent because of feeling threatened by another group member (Yalom, 1970). Whatever the reason, it is important that the member be encouraged to participate to help him feel more a part of the group. Enhancing feelings of belonging can frequently alleviate some of the member's fears and help him to feel more comfortable.

Given time, the other group members will generally bring the silent member into the verbal exchange (Toothman, 1978). If the more verbal members feel that they are risking, sharing, and perhaps exposing themselves, they may pressure the silent member into a more active role. They may think that the silent member is playing it safe (Levine, 1979) and feel that this is unfair. They are likely to want the silent member to not only share himself but also to react to what they have shared. Since the member is often silent because he fears judgment from the others, this interest and encouragement shown to him may be experienced as acceptance. There is another reason for leaving it up to the group members to facilitate the silent member's participation and this is to avoid reinforcing the authority role of the leader-therapist (Lifton, 1972). Actions taken by the leader-therapist to engage the quiet member may threaten the group. They may begin to wonder if she may also do something to cause them to feel uncomfortable. There are, however, some techniques that the leader-therapist may employ in attempting to involve the silent member that can be facilitative and constructive.

EYE CONTACT

Kell and Corts (1980) observed that a leader with "a keen interest in the participation of all the others in the group will maintain active eye contact" (p. 114). In any situation we are much more likely to talk if another person is looking directly at us when we speak. So to induce a quiet member to speak you can look directly at *him* when speaking to the whole group with the intention of encouraging him to respond. When an opportunity presents to say, "What does everyone think about that?," or, "How do people feel about that?," look at the quiet member as if you are expecting him to answer. It is easier for the member to respond in such a situation if you maintain eye contact than if you are glancing all around the group as you pose your question. Once the member is speaking it is easier to further facilitate his interaction with others.

AGREEMENT WITH OTHERS

If a member is struggling with one of the inhibiting factors mentioned previously, a first effort to bring him into the group may be to have him agree or disagree with a contribution by another member. To inquire, "Peter, do you agree with what Mary just said?," makes a very minor demand. Peter need only say yes or no. It is true that he is more likely to say yes in order to be left alone, but at least he has broken his barrier of silence by speaking. Breaking this barrier is the first big step to be taken toward becoming a participating member. The longer a member remains silent the more difficult it becomes for him to speak. Requesting Peter's agreement or disagreement also gives Peter the message that his thoughts on the subject are important and this in turn is likely to enhance his self-confidence.

ASKING FOR AN OPINION

To continue with the example of Peter above, once he has broken the barrier of silence by agreeing with another member you will want to follow up by getting a more individual response. You might try, "Peter, how do you feel about . . . ," or, "Peter, what is your opinion on. . ." This may put Peter on the spot, but with a caring and encouraging tone of voice you can give him the message that his feelings or opinions are important and both you and the group want to hear them. This may offer the encouragement or push he needs in order to feel a little safer and more comfortable in sharing his views. If he feels recognition and acceptance each time he speaks, this will increase the likelihood of him saying more and of eventually being able to participate spontaneously.

TAKING TURNS

The technique of going around the circle, with members in turn having their say, also works well in facilitating participation by the quiet member. It is not recommended as a continual way for the group to interact though, as it prohibits spontaneity and restricts interactions among the members. With this technique members become preoccupied with thinking of what they are going to say when it is their turn instead of listening to what is being said at the moment. It also takes away the opportunity for members to respond to one another immediately if it is not their turn, and thus important material is sometimes lost because the moment passes. However, it can be a very useful method to employ occasionally as a way of bringing each member into contact with the others or of encouraging participation when the group is very new or has run out of steam.

DIRECT QUESTIONING

If a member who usually participates appears withdrawn in a particular session, you might ask about his silence: "Robert, you usually share with us, but so far today you haven't said anything. Would you tell us why you are so quiet?" You need to be careful in phrasing your question in this instance because a closed-end question such as, "Robert, you are so quiet today. Is anything wrong?," may elicit only a negative response, leaving you no further ahead. So you want to ask the question in a format likely to elicit an explanation. His explanation can then be followed up with further questions or comments by yourself or other group members.

GROUP SILENCE

When the whole group is silent far greater discomfort is experienced by all who are present than when only one member is silent (Toothman, 1978). All groups will experience this type of total silence periodically and for different reasons. Silence can come at the resolution or conclusion of an issue or exchange leaving the group in a state of "Where do we go from here?" Conversely, silence may be the result of an unresolved issue with the members wondering, "What do we do now?" Perhaps some strong opposing views have been presented and the group reaches an impasse. Not knowing how to handle the conflict the members withdraw into silence. In another instance an individual may share a very intimate feeling or experience. Afraid to say the wrong thing or not knowing if they should say anything, the members choose to remain silent.

The leader-therapist must assess the reason for the silence, the stage of development the group is in, the membership, and the level of anxiety present to determine what would be the most facilitative intervention. This situation can be one of the most difficult moments for a leader-therapist. How she handles the situation will often depend solely on her own level of comfort or discomfort with the silence. Inexperienced leader-therapists tend to feel anxious during silence and are apt to overestimate its duration as well as feel a pressing need to do something to end it. This combination often leads them to take the initiative in intervening to break the silence.

A rule of thumb is that the most anxious person, whether member or leader-therapist, will make the move to end the silence. So if you, as leader-therapist, are feeling uncomfortable, you can be quite sure that some group members are feeling uncomfortable as well. The choice then becomes whether to wait for a member to intervene or whether to do so yourself. This decision will be based on your assessment of the immediate situation. Leaving it up to a group member to break the silence can sometimes be quite illuminating. It may be that what the member says is not at all what would have been expected under the circumstances. This may give everyone new information about the specific member, or the group in general, in terms of thoughts, feelings, and needs.

A different kind of silence can occur following a meaningful and moving interchange among a few or even all of the group members (Toothman, 1978). This type of silence is more comfortable and may be accompanied by some nonverbal exchanges while members relax and assimilate the experience. There is no tension evident and members give no indications of wanting to move on immediately.

TERMINATION

There are three primary types of termination that can occur in the life of a group. They are: (1) a group member stops coming to group, (2) the group, as an entity, ends because the contracted number of sessions have been completed, and (3) the staff member must end her role as leader-therapist in the group. There are also times when a group will terminate because of unplanned situational factors. For example, this could occur if there are too few clients available to maintain the group, or if the overall treatment program is suddenly changed. Such abrupt terminations do not allow for preplanning and can only be dealt with individually. The three primary types are discussed separately.

MEMBER TERMINATION

There can be several reasons why a member may stop coming to the group: he may be given an earlier discharge than was planned, he may discharge himself,

he may be dissatisfied with the group and so drops out, or he may be terminated because both he and the leader-therapist feel his planned goals have been
attained (Berne, 1966). Members who drop out usually do so because they
were not adequately prepared for the group, they do not feel the norms or goals
of the group are conducive to change, or they simply do not personally feel
comfortable in the group (Hansen, Warner, & Smith, 1976). Whenever a termination occurs, the occurrence needs to be addressed in the group, because the
absence will affect the overall dynamics of the group. In effect, if even one
member leaves the group, then the remaining members must reform into what
is basically a new group. This is especially true if the member has been an active
member and has played a significant role in the group.

In the situation where a member has been discharged it is likely that the leader-therapist has received advance notice, in which case she can pass this information on to the group. In doing so she should invite the members to express their
feelings about the member's discharge. The reactions of the remaining members are likely to vary, with some thinking they should leave also ("If he's ready
to go then so am I"), whereas others may fear being discharged before they feel
they are ready. It is therapeutic for the members to discuss these points and by
doing so move the group into functioning without the discharged member.

When it is known in advance that a member is to be discharged, it is a good
idea for the therapist to inform the group: "Does everyone know that Joe is
being discharged on Friday, so this will be his last group?" Making such an an-
nouncement allows the members to wish Joe well and for Joe to say anything
he has to say to the members. For example, he may want to comment on how
the group has helped him and to thank the members for their part in his progress. Another benefit of mentioning Joe's discharge to the group is to reinforce
the fact that clients do improve and in an indirect way offer hope and encouragement to the remaining members.

When a member drops out he may not inform anyone. He may just not appear
at the session. In this case the leader-therapist could ask if anyone knows where
the member is and if anyone would like to go and invite him to come to the
group. This is a good idea because on invitation the member may respond by
coming, and then the issue of his dropping out can be discussed with him. Sometimes the interactions with the other members prove useful to his deliberations
about leaving and are sufficient to cause him to change his mind and stay in the
group. Even if he declines the invitation to the session, showing concern for his
whereabouts can be received as a positive message by the remaining members
("Hey, they really care about people in this group"). The members should then be
given an opportunity to briefly discuss his decision to leave the group even
though he is not there. This allows the members to voice their feelings about his
absence and to explore and perhaps reaffirm their own need for the group.

GROUP TERMINATION

If the whole group is to be terminated because the contracted number of sessions is completed, the members should be reminded of this before the last

session ("Remember that next Friday is our last session so during the week try to think of anything you want brought up or discussed before the group ends"). This reminder jogs the members to think about the overall experience and encourages them to mention any issues or unfinished business that may be troubling them. It is then a good idea to begin the last group with a reference to it being the last session and invite the members to share any thoughts or feelings they have about unfinished business or the ending of the group. Try to plan this last session so there is a little time before its conclusion to talk about the overall experience, what members learned from it, and how they feel about the group being finished. It can also be very useful for your own learning to ask for suggestions and comments regarding the past sessions because this information may be of value in planning future groups. Drawing up a short evaluation form to be completed by each member at the close of the session can be useful. By having this prepared beforehand you will not forget any of the questions you wanted to ask.

LEADER-THERAPIST TERMINATION

Considering that a leader-therapist's absence from one session can be experienced as rejection by the members (Pollak, 1975), termination by a leader-therapist is a serious event. Many of the issues surrounding termination of a leader-therapist can be handled in much the same ways as were discussed for individual clients. The group should be informed of the termination as far in advance as possible with the reasons for the change being clearly stated. Members sometimes worry or think that the leader-therapist's leaving is their fault: they have not been a "good" group or the leader-therapist did not like them. Assurance should be given that the leader-therapist's leaving has nothing to do with the members, either individually or collectively.

It is not unusual for members to react negatively to the announced termination. Flapan and Fenchel (1987) note that cohesive groups and groups that have received news of the impending termination well in advance react more positively than do groups where these factors are not present. Members, especially those who have been attending for some time and have come to feel close to the leader-therapist, may feel they are being abandoned. Some acting-out behaviors may occur with members not showing up for group or being disruptive and uncooperative when present. It is important for the leader-therapist to acknowledge these feelings openly, but generally ("It's hard when people we have come to depend on leave us" . . . "I know it's hard when things change and you have to get used to a new person"). Try to give a positive message about the continuance of the group ("You all try so hard, I know that Mary is going to enjoy working with you"). Generally, making promises to visit the group or holding out hope of future contacts as a means of softening the parting is not recommended.

THE PSYCHOTIC MEMBER

Exclusion of the psychotic patient from psychotherapy groups as advocated by Yalom (1970) may be in the best interests of all. Levine (1979), however, suggests that chronic schizophrenics can be helped in homogeneous groups if the leader-therapist can accept their lower level of functioning. Task groups differ from psychotherapy groups and this writer believes the decision for inclusion or exclusion of a psychotic client should be based on assessment of the individual client. Several factors must be thoughtfully considered before making the decision. First and foremost is the severity of the psychosis. Clients who are violent or acutely disturbed need a brief period to settle down before further demands are made on them. Once the violent behavior is under control, inclusion in a task group may be appropriate. Being included can be experienced by the psychotic client as receiving attention, and this alone can have a tempering effect on his symptoms (Shapiro, 1978). Secondly, careful thought should be given to the type of group or activity in question. Different tasks or activities require different levels of functioning and participation. For example, role playing requires a high level of abstract thought and can be quite stimulating, whereas finger painting or drawing can accommodate psychotic thoughts and is more calming.

Most importantly, the leader-therapist needs to examine her own feelings and abilities in coping with a psychotic member in her group. If she feels nervous or unsure about handling the situation, then, for the benefit of everyone, she should not attempt to do so. The level of comfort and acceptance displayed by the rest of the group members toward the psychotic member will depend on the behavior of the leader-therapist and they will take their cues from her. If she is calm, accepting, orienting, and matter-of-fact with the disturbed member, they are likely to behave in the same way. Having a member who is more dysfunctional than they are can actually be a positive experience for the other members in that it gives them an opportunity to be helpful, perhaps feel more competent, and can sometimes offer a new perspective on their own problems. Naturally, it is easier to accommodate psychotic members if you have a co-leader. With the presence of two staff, if a member becomes particularly disturbed or decides to leave the group, there is a leader available to attend to the member individually while the other remains with the group.

Sitting beside the member, a technique used with monopolists (see above), also works well with individuals who are struggling with reality or who have poor impulse control. Your proximity allows you to orient the member or help him control his impulses without major disruption to the whole group. It gives you the opportunity to speak quietly to the member ("Wait until Mary has finished speaking" . . . "It's not your turn yet"). Even the interjection "Sh," with a finger to your lips, may be sufficient to prevent the member from constantly interrupting. This kind of limit setting assists the disturbed member with reality orientation by helping him become more aware of his own behavior. Soon the member may begin to catch himself by asking, "Am I interrupting?," or, "When is it my turn?" By being close you also have the opportunity of using touch as a gentle restrainer. A slight pressure on the arm may be sufficient to remind the individual that in group the members are expected to stay in their chairs. Also, by sitting beside the member you convey a message of support, of we-ness, rather than one of confrontation. If the leader-therapist is sitting across the group, she has to speak louder, perhaps gesture, or even move across the circle to catch the attention of the psychotic member. These behaviors can be very disruptive and divisive.

Kaplan (1986) describes a group which she believes promotes movement toward self-direction for severely incapacitated patients. She calls this group the "directive group." The group meets daily and is specifically for clients experiencing hallucinations, paranoia, catatonia, severe depression, organicity, hyperactivity, concrete thinking, or loose associations. She describes each session as having four distinct parts: (1) orientation and introductions, (2) warm-up activities, (3) selected activities, and (4) wrap-up. Reality-orienting activities are a major focus of the group, and include physical movements, relating to objects, and finally, interacting with other members. Because of the level of dysfunction of the members the co-leaders are instrumental in developing individual goals for the members. These include: (a) participation in the activities of each session, (b) verbal interaction with others around the common tasks, (c) punctuality and attendance for the full 45 minutes, and (d) initiation of relevant ideas for group activities (p. 478). Although Kaplan's experience with the directive group has been solely in a short-term setting, she believes it could be viable with the chronically ill as well.

APATHY

Apathy can be described as lack of interest or lack of motivation and may be observed in individual members or in the group as a whole. Leader-therapists are usually quick to recognize apathy by noticing some or all of the following attitudes and behaviors:

- Lack of interest in the task
- Low level of participation
- Reluctance to assume responsibility
- Decisions made without thought or discussion
- Failure to follow through on decisions
- Tedious discussion
- Loss of the point of the discussion
- Tardiness or absence of members
- Slouching and restlessness
- Frequent yawns

Apathy is a mood that can be contagious among the members and can present a difficult situation for the leader-therapist. In dealing with an apathetic group, determining the precipitating factors or the cause of the apathy is a first step. If the members are apathetic in their approach to a task there can be several possibilities: perhaps they do not like the task, cannot see the purpose of the task, feel inadequate to complete the task, or because of familiarity, are bored with the task. If one of these is thought to be a causative factor, then sometimes supplying more information, initiating a discussion of the problem, or changing the task can have a motivating effect. Speaking generally, members may appear apathetic because they feel overwhelmed with anxiety or depression, or they are bored, physically or mentally exhausted, or their interests at the moment are elsewhere. Sometimes it is just a bad day for the group, and conveying the message "this too shall pass" puts the least stress on everyone. At other times you might want to try to energize the group through some physical activity, warm-up exercises, or a fun event like a game.

CONFIDENTIALITY

The limits surrounding confidential material will vary depending on the nature of the group, but they remain a central ethical issue for all groups. It is the responsibility of the leader-therapist to inform all group members of the norms and limits concerning confidentiality in her facility. Information and material arising from inpatient groups is usually passed on to team members or is charted. Group members should be made aware of this routine. Leader-therapists must be careful not to make promises about confidential matters that they are unable to keep. For example, a member saying, "I'll tell you about this if you promise not to tell the doctor," can be an invitation to a no-win situation. By being honest and open you will build a trusting relationship with the members and, based on this, they will respect and understand the decisions you must make about material that is revealed in the group. Discussion needs to take place between the members and yourself to decide the confidential status of material shared in the group in regard to persons other than staff who are external to the group. Clients may come to the group from different units or wards and they are entitled to protection from group information being passed on to other residents.

SUMMARY

In this chapter the author has attempted to bring to the attention of the new leader-therapist certain problem situations that often occur in any group. It is believed that by being forewarned the leader-therapist can be somewhat prepared and better able to deal with the problems as they arise. The suggestions offered here are by no means the only ways of responding or dealing with the situations described. However, it is hoped that the ideas offered will serve to generate other solutions and prompt a problem solving approach in dealing with what can be experienced as difficult times in any group.

Some of the techniques presented in Chapter 7 are also useful in dealing with the effects of a monopolist, a nonparticipator, the member-to-leader-only dialogue, group silence, termination, apathy, and the psychotic member. It should be remembered, though, that each time one of these situations arises it will be a unique circumstance and must be responded to individually. There is no set response or intervention that guarantees success in a particular situation, and all outcomes using the suggestions offered will be in keeping with the approach and personality of the individual leader-therapist.

CHAPTER 9

Co-leadership

It takes two to speak the truth — one to speak and another to hear.
— HENRY DAVID THOREAU

Leader-therapists may work alone with a group or they may work in a dual leadership situation with a co-leader-therapist. Although little has been published as to the effectiveness of co-therapy in comparison with individual therapy (Rice, Razin, & Gurman, 1976), it is generally believed that co-therapy has value in promoting certain therapeutic outcomes (Rabin, 1967).

Different forms of co-therapy are reported in the literature with unique purposes ascribed to each. Possibly the most familiar and obvious use of co-therapy is in marital and family therapy where co-therapists of the opposite sex offer male and female models and simulate the family setting (Mullen & Sangiuliano, 1960; Russell & Russell, 1979). In short-term treatment of married couples, Markowitz and Kadis (1972) describe how the interactions of the co-therapists serve as "parental prototypes," which help the couple move toward maturity by dispelling their long-held perceptions and distortions of parental roles. Secondly, in co-therapy the adoption of opposing roles such as good-bad (MacLennan, 1965) and provocative-harmonizing (Yalom, 1970), used either deliberately or unwittingly, can at times be facilitative in meeting the myriad needs presented by group members. As a teaching method co-therapy provides a training situation where a trainee learning group therapy techniques is paired with a supervisor as co-therapist of the group. This situation requires a different relationship between the co-therapists from the egalitarian relationship that is usually recommended. Getty and Shannon (1969) advocate that co-therapists have similar levels of therapeutic experience, respect and accept each other, make joint decisions, share mutual responsibility, and enjoy equal opportunity for participation.

For the most part the literature addresses co-therapy in terms of advantages and disadvantages, with the former outweighing the latter (Yalom, 1970; Shapiro, 1978; Russell & Russell, 1979). In evaluating the use of co-therapy, Kottler (1983) says, "Many experienced leaders attribute their high morale, continuing growth, and avoidance of burn-out to their willingness to work in tandem with compatible colleagues" (p. 174). Although the advantages of co-leadership are noted by some to be of more benefit to the co-leaders than to the group members (Haley, 1976), others believe that the support inherent in co-leading has spin-off advantages for the group (Rosenbaum, 1973).

ADVANTAGES

BETTER GROUP COVERAGE

The old adage, "Two heads are better than one," has relevance for co-leaders. With two persons in the group listening and observing there is less chance of important material being missed and double the opportunity for awareness of process. If one leader becomes engrossed in an issue or interchange, the other leader, by observing the rest of the group, can pick up on the reactions of other members and deal with them when appropriate. If a member becomes upset or disturbed one leader can attend to this person while the co-leader monitors the functioning of the rest of the group (Corey & Corey, 1982; Hansen, Warner, & Smith, 1976). As well as supplying more manpower, two leaders offer the members variety and the benefit of their "combined insight and technical skill" (Mosey, 1986, p. 265).

COMPATIBILITY

Hansen, Warner, and Smith (1976) state that, "the presence of two counselors increases the possibility that every group member will be able to identify with at least one of the counselors" (p. 315). In any new meeting of two people there is the chance that one will not take to the other. So it is in groups. Sometimes a member will not like the leader, and similarly, there are times when a leader feels antipathy or has a particular aversion for a certain member. These circumstances may evolve through the distortions of transference and countertransference or because of ordinary incompatibility. In such situations it is possible for an antagonistic relationship to develop. Having a second leader who can interact comfortably with the member frequently diffuses what could become a potentially hostile situation. Partners who work well together will watch for signs of discord and intervene to the benefit of members, leaders, and member-leader interactions.

SHARING RESPONSIBILITIES

The role of a group leader can be a lonely and tiring experience. As sole leader-therapist one must be constantly alert, observing and attending to what is going on with and among all the group members. Simultaneously with attending to every nuance of speech and behavior, the leader-therapist must analyze the constantly changing situation to formulate her observations into meaningful constructs. Kottler (1983) gives a hypothetical but realistic description of the complex dynamics in a group and the infinite demands these put on the group leader.

I've got to press Sandra harder. She's slipping away with her typical game-playing manners. Perhaps I could . . . Ooops. Why is Rob squirming over in the corner? Did I hit one of his nerves? There go those giggling guys again. I better interrupt them before they begin their distracting jokes. Where was I? Oh yeah, I was formulating a plan to motivate Sandra. But she keeps looking to Jody and Melaine for approval. I must break that destructive bond between them. They keep protecting one another from any growth. And there's Cary acting bored again, dying for attention. I've got to ignore him and get back to the problem at hand. But what is the problem at hand? (p. 176)

Amusing though this may be to read, to work alone with such complex dynamics is an exhausting endeavor. Two leaders working cooperatively can minimize omissions and increase opportunities for interaction by sharing the responsibilities of leadership within the group sessions.

SUPPORT

Co-therapists serve as allies. They assume supportive roles, sharing the responsibilities and helping each other out of tricky situations that arise (Russell & Russell, 1979). This is not to imply a teaming up against the group but rather that together two leaders can offer more objectivity. If one leader is having difficulty understanding a member's point or getting his own point across to a member, the co-leader can often clarify by saying, "I think what Joe means is . . .", or, "Is what you are saying . . . ?" Thus a co-therapy format minimizes subjective reactions, misconceptions, and missed cues.

Group members can at times be very dependent and demanding. Co-therapists can share in shouldering these needs, or as Halperin (1987) puts it, "provide a needed measure of support" (p. 52). A co-leader who has been the primary facilitator in a particularly tense or active interval may want to take a brief emotional time-out to recoup her energies while the other monitors the group. Leader-therapists working alone do not have this option and may find the leadership role more taxing.

Every leader-therapist is prone to doubts and misgivings ("Should I have said that?" . . . "Was that the right thing to do?" . . . " How could I have handled that differently?"). The buildup of these questions and thoughts contributes to most leader-therapists having a need to talk or ventilate when the group is over. Co-therapists meet this need for each other. After a session they usually meet to discuss and analyze what happened, how things went, and how things could have been different. This postgroup interaction is a time for feedback, problem solving, sharing, and support.

CONTINUITY OF CARE

In the case where one leader must be absent due to illness, vacation, professional demands, or an emergency situation, the co-leader can carry on with the group, thus providing continuity. However, as with the absence of any member, the overall dynamics of the group will be affected. The remaining members often spend the first part of the group adjusting to and dealing with the absence, thus stalling the movement of the group. In comparison with the solution to the absence of a single leader (which could be pulling in a totally new leader-therapist) the disruption to the group in the case of an absent co-leader will be far less pronounced.

Group leaders will not always be in peak condition on group days. If one of the co-therapists happens to be feeling especially drained, run-down, or temporarily lethargic, the other is there to carry the load during that particular time or even for the session. In such a case it is best that the co-leader tells the group that she is having a bad day and because of this she may be quieter and less active than usual. This serves as good role modeling of openness for the members. It also conveys the message that even professionals are human and have down days. This can be comforting to members who feel inadequate in comparison with leaders whom they perceive as "having it all together."

ROLE MODELING AND ROLE PLAYING

Even a brief discussion of co-therapy would not be complete without mentioning the special advantages of this format in marital and family therapy. In marital therapy the co-leaders are usually of the opposite sex, sometimes husband and wife themselves, and therefore serve as role models for the couple (Russell & Russell, 1979). Having a co-leader of each sex also provides a balance of masculine and feminine support (Low & Low, 1975). Co-therapists work with families in much the same way, serving as both parental and spousal role models.

In a group the presence of two leaders, who are usually viewed as the authority figures, tends to simulate a family setting. This affords opportunities for more variety in the role playing of different family situations. A leader, by assuming the role of a family member, can interact with an individual in the group to role play and work out a troublesome situation. When one leader is involved in such role playing with a group member, the other leader is available to observe, comment, and give feedback. Role playing is an excellent way of involving members more actively in the group, of portraying situations more vividly, and of presenting opportunities for trying out new behaviors.

Often clients' problems stem from unsatisfactory and defective family situations. Their experience with relationships may be only ones of anger, conflict, and abuse, For these clients, observing co-therapists, who are two persons in relatively equal authoritative positions, accepting or working out their differences of opinions, feelings, and responses can be very enlightening. Viewing this process of acceptance and cooperation may also foster and facilitate the expression of differing feelings and opinions by the group members themselves (Gallogly & Levine, 1979).

TRAINING

Co-therapy is used as a format for training students or others in group and leadership skills. By experiencing complete immersion in the leadership role as a co-therapist, the trainee gains an intimate understanding of group dynamics and the role of the leader. The trained leader serves as a model for the trainee and the latter feels safe in experimenting with interventions and techniques as she knows immediate help and support are available. Although Yalom (1970) cautions against a co-therapy arrangement between persons of unequal status, it is believed that the training situation is a viable exception (Corey & Corey, 1982). This situation does require some special attention, especially from the leader-trainer. The acceptance of the trainee as a co-leader, in the full sense of that role, will depend on how the student presents herself or is presented to the group by her co-leader. It should be stated, preferably by the student herself, that she is a student or trainee and that she will be participating in the group as co-therapist. By announcing her role in this manner she is asking the group to treat her more as a leader than as a student. If her student status is emphasized there is a chance the group members will focus all their attention on the "real" leader, turning the situation into a one-leader rather than a co-leader group.

Supervision, which should occur after the group, is where the trained leader needs additional skill. For her to gain feedback for herself and to ensure a two-way dialogue during the postgroup discussion, she must create a sense of sharing and an environment of equality. By creating a cooperative atmosphere it is anticipated that the student will feel encouraged to express her feelings about the co-therapist relationship along with her impressions and thoughts about the group. This mutual sharing allows both participants to learn from the experience. In addressing the issue of training Williams (1976) states his preference for having students learn the skills of leadership by being co-leaders themselves and receiving supervision outside the group. He believes this method avoids tensions and prevents role confusion.

DISADVANTAGES

The disadvantages of the co-therapy situation have been called "hazards" (Yalom, 1970) and "dangers" (Shapiro, 1978) and are based mainly on the nature and quality of the co-leader relationship. Kottler (1983) says, "Unless partners can work as a complementary team, much group time can be wasted in power plays, bickering and mutual sabotage" (p. 178). He describes devastating situations that can occur in groups as a result of competitiveness between co-leaders. Leaders competing with each other invariably involve the group by trying to enlist members' support in their cause or position, resulting in group members taking sides. Splitting of the group can also emerge if one leader is challenged by a group member(s) and her co-leader supports the challenge. A nasty situation can arise if the leader has been harboring negative feelings or reactions and uses this situation of challenge as an opportunity to unload her own previously unexpressed feelings onto her co-leader. Competition between co-leaders is likened to the conflicts between parents who are competing for their children's affection.

Another circumstance with inherent problems for co-leaders is the situation where one leader has a more dominant personality and a strong need for control. The dominant partner will tend to overshadow her co-leader and the advantages of co-leadership will be lost. This almost always has a negative effect on the group. Pacing is yet another potential area for problems. Co-leaders need to be able to "lead" at relatively equivalent speeds in order to feel comfortable and be able to keep the group moving in a consistent manner (Shapiro, 1978). They each need to respect and trust their co-leader's competence to prevent undermining and to ensure that each will place value on the interventions made by the other. If co-leaders respect and trust each other's judgment, then when differences do occur they can be dealt with in a constructive manner.

Most of the dangers of co-therapy can be avoided through the careful selection of a co-leader. However, a leader-therapist may not always have the prerogative of selecting her co-leader. In this case it is doubly important for the co-therapists to hold informational discussions before the group to acquaint each other with their individual approaches, methods, preferences, and ways of leading. This can be a time to identify differences that could lead to problems and to work out methods for handling such problems should they crop up in the group session. Time should also be spent in planning the group so that the co-therapists know who is going to do what, and when (Mosey, 1986).

THE CO-THERAPY RELATIONSHIP

Most authors agree that the relationship between the two leader-therapists is the crucial factor in effective co-therapy (Gallogly & Levine, 1979; Russell & Russell, 1979; Shapiro, 1978). Williams (1976) delineates several issues requiring attention and consideration by both partners in order to ensure an effective co-therapy relationship. These are presented here in part.

COMMUNICATION

To say that co-leaders need to communicate may seem elementary, but the importance of this point needs to be emphasized. In the busy and pressured work environments of most therapists it can be difficult to schedule time, both before and after group, for talking together. Yet the need for such discussions is paramount for the co-leader relationship to be sustained. A brief meeting before the group enables the leaders to make contact and check out how the other is feeling, both within themselves and about the impending session. This contact also allows the leaders to refresh their memories about any pertinent events or incidents from the last group and to establish plans and goals for the ensuing one. Communication between the leaders will also occur during the session and can serve two purposes: to make the therapists appear more human, and to role model proficient communication methods. The postgroup discussion between the co-leaders is crucial and will be presented separately.

The fact that co-leaders are usually professional therapists or counselors does not mean that they will always know the intentions of the other or send clear messages (Figure 9-1). It is essential that any communication between the co-therapists is made clear and understood. If a co-leader does not understand a statement or an action taken by her partner, she should immediately try to clarify the meaning, whether the communication occurs pregroup, during group or postgroup. During the session, such efforts at clarification serve as good role models for the group members. It gives them the message, "If you don't understand something, you ask." It can also be true that if the co-leader missed the meaning of what her partner said, it is quite likely that some members missed it as well, and by seeking clarification the co-leader will help clarify the issue for everyone.

POSTGROUP ANALYSIS

The co-leaders need to meet after each session to share their thoughts and feelings about the group, to discuss and analyze the process, and to note any sig-

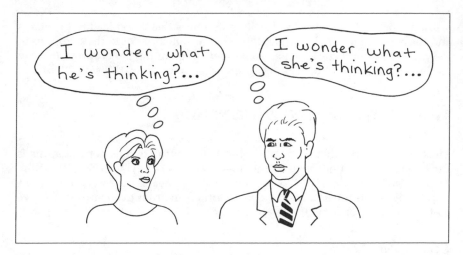

Figure 9-1. Lack of communication in co-therapists.

nificant dynamics. A point should be made to examine the participation of each member so that this information can be relayed back to the appropriate team members. As a result of events or incidents in the session, plans may be made as to how to deal with certain members or situations in future groups. It is also essential during this postgroup analysis for the co-leaders to discuss their interactive relationship, focusing on such questions as: Were their interventions compatible? In what instances did they agree or disagree, and were these handled to their mutual satisfaction? What changes or adaptations need to be made in their ways of relating, either to each other, or to the members? In short, how well did they work together?

ASSETS AND LIMITATIONS

An effective co-therapy team is based on the enhancement of each other's assets in concert with downplaying (rather than exploiting) each other's limitations. Giving each other positive feedback on behaviors and interventions is conducive to building self-confidence and a cooperative working relationship. This is not to say that negative aspects should be ignored, but by creating a positive, respectful atmosphere the negatives are more easily given and more readily received. Differences and disagreements should be confronted, but with a constructive ("What should we do about it?") approach rather than a finger-pointing ("What are you going to do about it?") stance.

COMPETITIVE TEMPTATIONS

There is no place for grandstanding or one-upmanship in a co-leader team. The success of co-therapy depends on a "we" approach and, as noted earlier, any competitive behaviors between the leaders are destructive to both the co-leader relationship and the group. Even the simple act of leader A assuming responsibility for introducing both leaders to the group can give the impression of leader A having a senior or more important role in the group than leader B. It should be remembered that the prominence gained by one leader over the other through competitive behavior will cost in terms of the ultimate effectiveness of the co-therapy method. The willingness and ability of leader-therapists to work together as a team is the cornerstone for the success of co-therapy.

PROFESSIONAL DIFFERENCES

Leader-therapists who endorse widely differing theoretical beliefs, such as the behavioral and analytical, are prone to have more difficulty working out a compatible co-leader relationship than will therapists coming from the same or similar theoretical positions.

This should be kept in mind in the selection or pairing of co-therapists. Co-therapists sharing similar theoretical approaches can more easily and quickly tune in to the intents of and purposes of the other at any given time. Because of this compatible awareness they are more likely and able to be supportive and helpful to each other. In the event of a crisis they feel more comfortable and confident in predicting dependable ways in which the other will respond. Now, having made a point of co-leaders sharing similar theoretical backgrounds, it should be clarified that co-therapists practicing different theoretical methods can certainly work together and indeed frequently complement each other very effectively. As long as they understand and accept the diversities of the other's techniques, problems can usually be avoided.

SUPERVISION

The type and degree of supervision required by co-therapists depends on the nature of the co-leader relationship. If it is a training situation and one of the co-leaders is a student, the senior leader-therapist will likely serve as supervisor. If the co-leaders share equal but limited leadership experience they might want and need to meet with a senior person as supervisor on a regular basis. For more experienced leader-therapists, occasional meetings with a supervisor to focus on the co-therapy relationship can be effective. Certainly, if there are problems in the co-therapy relationship, outside consultation should be sought as soon as possible.

RESOLVING FEELINGS AND CONFLICTS

Although sharing feelings is part of communicating, it is such an important part that it requires a separate heading. It is imperative that co-therapists be honest in telling each other how they feel. Holding back feelings of anger, resentment, disappointment, or hurt will definitely affect their interrelating and hence the total therapeutic endeavor. Naturally, they should not choose to air their peeves during the group. However, an occasional disagreement between the leaders is inevitable and can be healthy both in resolving their differences and in role-modeling problem resolution. It helps members realize that having a disagreement is a normal occurrence in a relationship, that it does not promote a crisis, and can be resolved by talking and sharing feelings. For intense feelings and disagreements the leaders should wait for their postgroup discussion to talk and work things out. If they are unable to resolve an issue through discussion, then this would be an occasion to seek outside help in the form of supervision.

Therapists should realize when entering into a co-leader relationship that there are likely to be some areas of conflict or disagreement. If they are prepared for the inevitability of such instances, their reactions will be more restrained and their outlook more positive when the first conflict arises.

PRACTICING WHAT THEY PREACH

This last point, made by Williams (1976), really speaks for itself. Leader-therapists are constantly urging and encouraging group members to interact, express their feelings, be open and honest, and direct and clear in communicating with others. It seems only fair, if they are asking their clients to do this, that they be prepared to practice what they preach.

Being part of a co-therapy team can be a gratifying experience. It offers opportunities for learning, skill development, and personal growth. Frequently, co-therapists are from different disciplines bringing varied backgrounds, methods, and ideas to the relationship. Combined with recognition, respect, and acceptance, such differences can enhance the co-therapy process. Most importantly, the partners must always bear in mind that the relationship needs careful attention and nurturing for it to be a truly collaborative effort.

SUMMARY

Assuming the role of co-therapist can be an exciting and rewarding experience and one that should be approached with openness and cooperation. Whether your co-therapist is of the same sex or the same profession as yourself, has equal training and skill, or shares the same theoretical approach, he or she should receive your respect, support, and acceptance. As in any relationship, in a co-therapy relationship you need to work together in an atmosphere of compatibility and shared responsibility. Approached in a spirit of exploration and learning, the co-therapy experience can be very stimulating. Defining and redefining the relationship can be done through frequent communication and discussion, analysis of interactions, supervision, recognition and resolution of differences, avoidance of competition, and by emphasizing each others' assets.

Having a co-therapist takes some of the pressure off you to be all things to all people. It provides for emergencies by offering continuity of care and allows for variety in role playing. Co-therapists bring different points of view to the group setting and those of opposite sex serve as male and female role models. Taking advantage of the opportunity to act as a co-therapist can be a motivating and inspirational experience.

CHAPTER 10

Observations and Analysis

Nothing that man possesses is more precious than his awareness.

— ROBERT DEROPP

Any analysis of a group should contain observations and information about the two components of a group: content and process. Since initially group members do not concern themselves directly with the process, they will focus on content, which would include the task and what is being said. It is the role of the leader-therapist to be aware of and monitor both components. You will want to check to see if the content is appropriate to the goals and if the process is moving the group toward achieving these goals. Your observations and sensitivity to the dynamics are crucial to following and understanding the meaning of the process. This will enable you to diagnose issues and problems early and so facilitate dealing with them more effectively. Observation guidelines can be helpful in emphasizing certain factors that need scrutinizing in order to analyze your group. Some of these, mentioned by Pfeiffer and Jones (1972), are: the members, verbal and nonverbal participation, influence, atmosphere, and feelings.

WHAT TO LOOK FOR

MEMBERS

Any person who is part of a group, be it a social or therapeutic group, wants to feel that he belongs. He wants to feel accepted and included. It is up to the leader-therapist to think about each member in terms of this aspect of the group experience. Does each member feel that he or she is a part of the group? Bob is pretty quiet; is he feeling left out? No one seems to respond to Mary; is she being ignored? John just pushed his chair back; is something bothering him? Observations like these need to be checked out and analyzed in the context of the total process. In keeping with these observations you will want to be alert to "subgrouping". Sometimes two or three members will form a clique and, deliberately or not, will behave in ways that exclude the others. This can foster resentments and may even be the cause of some members not wanting to return to the next group session. A similar, but perhaps more divisive situation, is when you have a couple of subgroups present who are opposed or in conflict with each other. The subgroups may have formed outside the group during ward activities or leisure time and although they do not pertain to the group per se, the members have brought their peeves along with them. If you sense such opposition or hostility among members it is crucial that you facilitate some discussion around the issue in an effort to resolve or dissipate the antagonism. Otherwise such subgroupings can have a very deleterious effect on the whole group experience. Make an effort to always be aware of which members are "in" the group and which are "outside." If you perceive that a member is outside, try to figure out why. It is possible it is his own choice, but it may be that certain dynamics occurring in the group, like subgrouping, are a factor in preventing his involvement. In the latter case a supportive intervention may be required to involve the member and help him to feel more a part of the group.

Observing and actually charting members' contributions in terms of membership roles (see Chapter 12) can be useful in obtaining an overall view of the group. Another way is to focus on more discreet behaviors (e.g., Who interrupts? Who fidgets? Who is talkative? Who is silent? Who questions? Who answers? Who is open? Who is closed?, etc.). Discerning these roles assists in your analysis of the process. For example, if members are constantly being interrupted you might ask yourself (or the group): "Is anybody listening?"

Everyone's behavior changes from time to time. Each session is a new experience for the members just as each day is a new day. Thoughts change, feelings change, the group composition may change, so it is a good idea to focus your observations and initial questions on finding out how each person is feeling. An early check like this can often tap into and ward off the possibility of problems arising later in the session. If Tom appears upset or angry it is better to deal with it at the beginning of the group, rather than risk that his feelings will affect the whole group's experience negatively. Similarly, if an individual seems to be especially high, some recognition and an inquiry into this state is appropriate. Vigilance is required throughout the session in order to be aware of affective changes in any of the members. The main point is to watch for changes in behaviors, especially abrupt changes, and then, through checking directly or making further observations, try to establish causes and meanings.

VERBAL AND NONVERBAL PARTICIPATION

Observing the verbal participation of the group members is quite straightforward, but picking up on the nonverbal messages requires a sensitive general awareness. It means constantly scanning the group watching for changing facial expressions and postures, listening for changes in voice tones, and being alert to gestures. All of these will contribute to your general analysis of what is going on in the group. In terms of verbal interactions a continual questioning of what you hear and observe will facilitate your analysis. Who talks to whom and how much? Is the seating arrangement affecting participation? Do the verbal members tend to take over the group? Are the quiet members squelched when they try to participate? What are the shifts and changes in participation? Do the high participators become quiet and the quiet members suddenly become talkative? If so, why? Did something specific happen that should be dealt with? Who keeps the ball rolling and how does the rest of the group react to this member? Are they relieved, resistive, compliant, annoyed, or interested? The behaviors of individual members, such as compulsive talking, scapegoating, and attention seeking, can impede the participation of others. Always consider that each member's participation has the potential for blocking, encouraging, or affecting in other ways the rest of the group. The questions and answers that you generate, either within yourself or from the members, will influence your analysis and direct the types of interventions you make.

Content is also a factor in participation. Members' likes or dislikes of the task will determine to a great extent the degree of their involvement. Your observations will help you analyze the task as being appropriate or inappropriate for the group at this time. Is it too easy, too complex, not of interest to these particular members, or just not relevant in the context of the group today? Your analysis of the situation may suggest that a change or adaptation of the task is in order. What about the discussion? Is it superficial with the members skirting issues? Or are they honestly grappling with their problems? Sometimes making a contribution to the content by way of sharing a personal experience of your own can affect the affective nature of the discussion. A good idea? Analyze and decide.

INFLUENCE

A member may be an active participator but have very little influence in the group. He may have a lot to say, but in spite of this he is basically ignored by the other group members. Another member may say very little, but when he does speak he commands the attention of the whole group. This member is said to have influence. Members with influence frequently emerge as leaders. Leader-therapists, of course, have a strong influence on the group and must be careful to always use it wisely. Their status affords them the ultimate power in the group, but exercising this power, except under exceptional circumstances, without consulting with or explaining to the group, can be a destructive maneuver.

The group as a whole usually has more influence than any individual member (Mosey, 1986), but a particularly powerful person is capable of influencing the whole group. This can present problems if the influence is not thought to be productive ("a bad influence"). A member may be awarded power by his status alone, and because the other members assume a he-knows attitude, they are reluctant to disagree or try to promote their own ideas. This usually calls for a gatekeeping intervention by the leader-therapist to facilitate participation by the other members.

In analyzing your group you will want to determine how and why the members or just certain members are being influenced. Three major ways of responding positively to influence are described by Mosey (1986). They are presented here as ways the group as a whole might respond but hold true for the responses of individual members. First, the group may respond to influence because they see the possibility of achieving desired outcomes. This is like jumping on the bandwagon to reap rewards. Second, the group or some members may want to stay on good terms with the person of influence to ensure that they are in concert with what they perceive is likely to be the winning side. Lastly, the members may genuinely agree with the ideas and propositions of an individual and so feel inclined and comfortable in responding positively. Influential members can be key figures in your group and need special heed. In observing the group or certain members being influenced, the analysis should focus on the effects of the influence to determine if the results are productive or destructive for the well-being of all the members. Influential members can be key figures in your group.

ATMOSPHERE

Most people have experienced being part of a group where the tension has been "so thick you could cut it with a knife." Tension of this severity usually results from long-standing rifts or recognized differences and is not likely to occur often in a therapeutic group. What can occur though, if there has been a particularly upsetting incident such as a violent act on the treatment unit, is that the group members may collectively feel nervous and tense. Other possible tension-producing events are new members joining the group, conflicts among or between individuals, and members experiencing severe emotional upsets. It can be beneficial to check with the ward or unit staff prior to the session to find out if there have been any recent disturbing incidents.

Conversely, at another time you may find that the members of the group are feeling high. Some may be excited in anticipation of day or weekend passes, others because they are having a good day, and still others as a symptom of their illness. Whatever the reason the elevated spirits are often contagious, making it difficult for the members to focus on the task or discussion at hand. Having observed the rising mood you then need to decide, based on your analysis of what is going on, what plan of action you will take. For example, you might decide that doing a few exercises may help the members dissipate some of their excess energy and enable them to settle down. Checking the prevailing atmosphere in the group is similar to determining the mood and affect of a client in a mental status examination. Changes in the atmosphere, especially abrupt ones, usually are indicative of something going on among the members. Observe it. Check it. Analyze it.

As mentioned elsewhere, the leader plays a key role in establishing the atmosphere of any group. If you are down and the group seems down, recognizing this similarity is probably the first step in your analysis of the dynamics. Something else to be aware of is that all members do not enjoy the same affective atmosphere. Some will prefer a totally congenial atmosphere and will quickly attempt to suppress any conflict or expression of negative feelings. Others seem to thrive on disagreement and may actively provoke or annoy their fellow members to "stir things up a bit." It is the responsibility of the leader-therapist to be sensitive to these differences, observe their effects, and after analyzing the options take whatever action is felt to be necessary.

FEELINGS

When we refer to a person with a psychiatric illness we talk about him having "emotional" problems. In many cases the emotional problem stems from the person's controlling his emotions through defense mechanisms, such as repression or suppression (Kaplan & Sadock, 1985) Often the task in a therapy group is designed to purposely precipitate the sharing of emotions by the members as a method of helping them learn how to express their feelings. For some this will be much more difficult than for others. Feelings are also frequently generated by the interactions among members during group sessions. In all instances of members expressing emotions your observations should focus on the quality of the experience for the member. Are the other members supportive? Is caring shown? How intense are the feelings? An analysis of the situation should tell you when and if you should intervene. Watch for a buildup of emotions in a member. If feelings are expressed at the time of first awareness they can usually be expressed in a relatively calm way, whereas after buildup there is a risk of a more explosive reaction. You may start to think of yourself as a broken record, always asking questions like, "How do you feel?" or "Mary, you seem to be feeling [sad, angry, frustrated . . .]." However, such comments help members to focus on and think about how they really are feeling and their answers help you to check out your observations and speculations. With time, and your role modeling, members will hopefully begin to check and verify feelings they suspect in one another("Mary, did what I just said upset you?"). One of the terminal goals, of course, is for the members to transfer these skills of recognizing, expressing, and checking out feelings to their relationships outside the therapeutic setting. In the meantime it is essential that you continue to monitor the feeling states of your members and facilitate the expression of feelings as they arise.

Monitoring is done, for the most part, by observing facial expressions, gestures, voice tone, change in posture, and other nonverbal cues. For example, if a participating member suddenly withdraws into silence you will want to find out the reason for this abrupt change in his behavior. Did someone say something that angered him? Maybe a comment precipitated his recall of an upsetting incident. Is he feeling ignored by the other members? Did he just remember that his weekend pass was cancelled and has this squelched his enthusiasm and interest in the group? If the feelings of this member are not brought out into the open his withdrawal can have a negative effect on the other members. Another member may think he said something "wrong" or upsetting so he may also pull back. Other members, uncomfortable with the silence of two members, may decide that the two members withdrew because they did not like what was going on in the group. To remedy this the rest of the group takes off in an entirely new or different direction. By this time the group is floundering, all the members are feeling pretty anxious, and little is being accomplished. All this is by way of emphasizing how watching for and identifying possible pent-up feelings serves as both a facilitative and preventive measure.

INTERACTION PROCESS ANALYSIS

A more formal method of observation and analysis has been formulated by Bales (1951, 1970). He presents a detailed, in-depth, but in its entirety, a rather complicated method of analyzing interactions based on task and maintenance issues. For a comprehensive examination of Bales's method the reader is referred to his books as only an overview of his selected categories is presented here. The term *process analysis* differentiates his type of analysis from methods of "content analysis." As shown in Figure 10-1, there are 12 categories of interaction which are broken down into four subsets. The first six categories are reciprocal or opposite to the second six categories. When observing a group Bales believes it is difficult to evaluate both process and content inclusively. How-

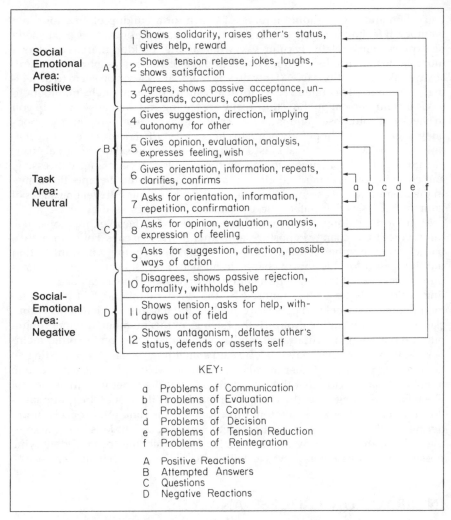

Social
Emotional   1   Shows solidarity, raises other's status,
Area: A   gives help, reward
Positive   2   Shows tension release, jokes, laughs,
                       shows satisfaction
                   3   Agrees, shows passive acceptance, un-
                       derstands, concurs, complies

                   4   Gives suggestion, direction, implying
                B   autonomy for other
                   5   Gives opinion, evaluation, analysis,
                       expresses feeling, wish
Task   6   Gives orientation, information, repeats,
Area: clarifies, confirms   a b c d e f
Neutral   7   Asks for orientation, information,
                       repetition, confirmation
                C 8   Asks for opinion, evaluation, analysis,
                       expression of feeling
                   9   Asks for suggestion, direction, possible
                       ways of action

                   10 Disagrees, shows passive rejection,
Social-   formality, withholds help
Emotional   D 11 Shows tension, asks for help, with-
Area: draws out of field
Negative   12 Shows antagonism, deflates other's
                       status, defends or asserts self

KEY:

a   Problems of Communication
b   Problems of Evaluation
c   Problems of Control
d   Problems of Decision
e   Problems of Tension Reduction
f   Problems of Reintegration

A   Positive Reactions
B   Attempted Answers
C   Questions
D   Negative Reactions

Figure 10-1. Bales interaction process analysis. Source: From R. Bales, *Interaction Process Analysis: A Method for the Study of Small Groups.* Reprinted by permission of University of Chicago Press. © 1950 by University of Chicago. All rights reserved.

ever, he also believes that in evaluating the "how" of the communications the observer can obtain important information about the members and what is happening in the group. For example, if you used Bales's categories and found that a member's interactions always fell in the D categories, you would want to explore these findings with the member to determine the basis for his consistent "negative reactions." Or if you had noticed some conflicts or uneasiness in the group but had been unable to fix its origin, analyzing the observation forms could be helpful. In doing this, should you find a member who always appeared to function in the "disagrees" category, you would be interested in determining if this member's behavior was affecting the group in a negative way. The next step would be to observe the reactions of the other members to this individual and analyze the overall interactive process.

ADAPTATION OF FORMS

Bales's definitions of the 12 categories are very complex by virtue of being broken down into various subtypes. Some of the categories are almost too broad to be useful in this original form. For instance, in the second category, "jokes," and, "shows satisfaction," could be two very different and opposite types of interaction. As you use these interaction forms and become more skilled in your ability to observe and record you may find that some of the categories are not relevant to your populations or types of groups. It will be of benefit, then, for you to adapt the forms to more accurately reflect the process and purpose of your particular group. If you should do this it is important to have a clear understanding of the meaning of any new categories. For example, if you are using the member role evaluation form (shown in Chapter 12, Figure 12-2), you may find that the category "information/opinion giver" does not accurately reflect an individual's sharing of personal feelings within the group. Since personal sharing is considered to be an important aspect of therapeutic groups, you may wish to include a category under "individual roles" to cover such contributions. You would then need to formulate a definition to define the types of contributions or comments that would be evaluated as "personal sharing" or whatever descriptor you select for the new category. It is possible that you may want to have separate forms for task groups and discussion groups. Since the member role evaluation form primarily reflects the kinds of interactions that occur in task groups, it may not be as useful when observing discussion groups. Whatever form you use or devise, make sure that you have clear descriptors formulated for each of your categories.

Both the informal and the formal methods of observation presented so far look primarily at the contributions and interactions of individual members. Although it is possible to examine the completed forms from these observational methods and obtain some measure of a group profile, Dimock (1985a) presents a method of surveying several dimensions of the whole group. By using his survey with the same group over several sessions, one is able to obtain an idea of the group's development over time. Dimock's survey is presented in Table 10-1.

INTERACTION DIAGRAMS

Diagrams such as those shown in Figure 10-2 and 10-3 are frequently used to capture a picture of the interaction process of a group. Based on the sociometric approach (Nixon, 1979) such interaction diagrams are similar to sociograms except they do not include the interpersonal sentiment of the interactions. Howe

Table 10-1. SURVEY OF GROUP DEVELOPMENT

For each area, place an X in the box that most nearly describes the group.

1. **UNITY** (Degree of unity, cohesion, or "we-ness")

☐ Group is just a collection of individuals or subgroups; little group feeling.

☐ Group is very close and there is little room or need felt for other contacts and experience.

☐ Some group feeling; unity stems more from external factors than from real friendship.

☐ Strong common purpose and spirit based on real friendships; group usually sticks together.

2. **SELF-DIRECTION** (The group's own motive power)

☐ Little drive from anywhere, either from members or leader.

☐ Domination from a strong single member, a clique, or leader.

☐ Group has some self-propulsion but needs considerable push from leader.

☐ Initiation, planning, executing, and evaluating comes from total group.

3. **GROUP CLIMATE** (The extent to which members feel free to be themselves)

☐ Climate inhibits good fun, behavior, and expression of desire, fears, and opinions.

☐ Members freely express needs and desires; joke, tease, and argue to detriment of the group.

☐ Members express themselves but without observing interests of total group.

☐ Members feel free to express themselves but limit expression to total group welfare.

4. **DISTRIBUTION OF LEADERSHIP** (Extent to which leadership roles are distributed among members)

☐ A few members always take leader roles; rest are passive.

☐ Many members take leadership but one or two are continually followers.

☐ Some of the members take leader roles but many remain passive followers.

☐ Leadership is shared by all members of the group.

5. **DISTRIBUTION OF RESPONSIBILITY** (Extent to which responsibility is shared among members)

☐ Everyone tries to get out of jobs.

☐ Many members accept responsibilities but do not carry them out.

☐ Responsibility is carried by a few members.

☐ Responsibilities are distributed among and carried out by nearly all members.

6. **PROBLEM SOLVING** (Group's ability to think straight, make use of everyone's ideas, and decide creatively about its problems)

☐ Not much thinking as a group; decisions made hastily, or group lets member-leader or leader do most of the thinking.

☐ Some thinking as a group but not yet an orderly process.

☐ Some cooperative thinking but group gets tangled up in pet ideas or prejudices of a few; confused movement toward good solutions.

☐ Good pooling of ideas and orderly thought; everyone's ideas are used to reach final plan.

7. **METHOD OF RESOLVING DISAGREEMENTS WITHIN GROUP** (How does group work out disagreements?)

☐ Group follows lead of member-leader or waits for leader to resolve disagreements.

☐ Compromises are effected by each subgrouping giving up something.

☐ Strongest subgroup dominates through a vote and majority rule.

☐ Group as a whole arrives at a solution that satisfies all members and is better than any single suggestion.

8. **MEETS BASIC NEEDS** (Extent to which group gives a sense of security, achievement, approval, recognition, and belonging)

☐ Group experience adds little to the meeting of most members' needs.

☐ Group experience contributes substantially to basic needs of most members.

☐ Group experience contributes to some degree to basic needs of most members.

☐ Group contributes substantially to basic needs of all members.

9. **VARIETY OF ACTIVITIES**

☐ Little variety in activities — stick to same things.

☐ Considerable variety in activities; try out new activities.

☐ Some variety in activities.

☐ Great variety in activities; continually trying out new ones.

10. **DEPTH OF ACTIVITIES** (Extent to which activities are gone into in such a way that members can use full potentialities — skill, creativity)

☐ Little depth in activities — just scratching the surface.

☐ Considerable depth in activities; members able to utilize some of their ability.

(continued)

Table 10-1 *(continued)*

10. **DEPTH OF ACTIVITIES** *(continued)*

☐ Some depth but members are not increasing their skills.

☐ Great depth in activities; members find each a challenge to develop their abilities.

11. **LEADER-MEMBER RAPPORT** (Relations between the group and the leader) Fill in percentage who are:

☐ Antagonistic or resentful.

☐ Friendly and interested; attentive to leader's suggestions and behavior.

☐ Indifferent toward leader; friendship neither sought nor rejected; noncommunicative.

☐ Intimate; open and sharing, with strong rapport.

12. **ROLE OF THE LEADER** (Extent to which the group is centered about the leader, his needs and interests)

☐ Activities, discussion, and decisions revolve about interests, desires, and needs of the leader.

☐ Leader acts as stimulator; suggests ideas or other ways of doing things; helps group find ways of making own decisions and solving problems.

☐ Group looks to leader for suggestions and ideas. Leader decides, when member gets in a jam.

☐ Leader stays out of discussion and makes few suggestions of things to do; lets members carry the ball themselves.

13. **STABILITY**

☐ High absenteeism and turnover influences group a great deal.

☐ Some absenteeism and turnover with minor influence on group.

☐ High absenteeism and turnover influences group growth very little.

☐ Low absenteeism and turnover; group very stable.

Source: Adapted from H. G. Dimock (1985a), *How to observe your group* (2nd ed.). Guelph, Ont., Canada, University of Guelph.

and Schwartzberg (1986) suggest a method of combining the two, by "marking the lines of the sociogram with letters keyed to Bales's categories" (p. 125). However, this method would place overwhelming demands on the observer when one considers the fluency with which members generally interact. Interaction diagrams are useful in showing the frequency of interactions and who speaks to whom. They show the diversity and direction of participation. Does Sally always talk to John? Does Mary usually speak to the group as a whole and

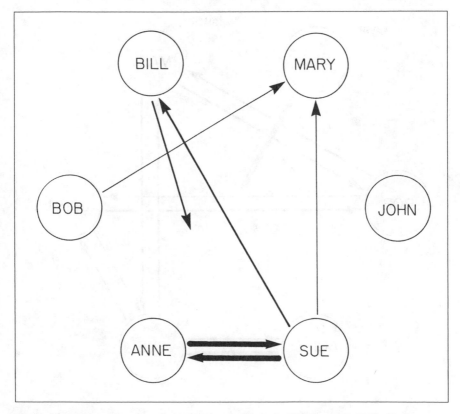

Figure 10-2. Interaction diagram early in session (see also Figures 10-3–10-5). Circles represent group members. Thin lines depict one communication. Medium lines depict two to three communications. Thick lines depict more than three communications.

to no one in particular? Do Ann and Don always talk to each other? To be aware of such patterns of relatedness can be informative and helpful in analyzing the process in a group (Dimock, 1985b).

Another way in which interaction diagrams are valuable, and this is demonstrated in Figures 10-2 and 10-3, is in showing changes in the interaction process of the group. When observations are made at different times in the group one can observe if the interactions are the same or different in the two samples. The maximum time duration for noting the interactions in your group should be 3 to 5 minutes. Recording over a longer interval does not afford an opportunity for comparison and usually results in such a mass of lines that a clear picture does not emerge.

Interaction diagrams are usually completed by an observer sitting outside the group because it is inhibiting and disruptive to have a person within the group noting each time a member speaks. Each time a person speaks an arrow is drawn from the speaking member to the member to whom the remark was

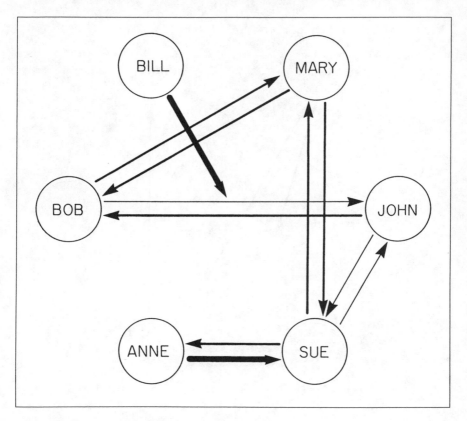

Figure 10-3. Interaction diagram late in session.

directed. Further remarks are noted by adding slash marks. A member speaking to the whole group is represented by an arrow drawn from the member to the center of the group only. For purposes of clarity lines of differing thickness have been used here to indicate the number of communications (see symbolic key, Figure 10-2).

On examining the interaction diagram in Figure 10-2 we might think about the following: Anne and Sue talk to each other frequently. Bill mostly speaks to the group as a whole and it appears that only Sue responds to him. Are Sue and Bob making an effort to include Mary in the discussion? If so, she does not respond. And what about John? He is not participating.

Our second view of the group is depicted in Figure 10-3. This diagram represents the interaction over a 3-minute period 10 minutes before the group is scheduled to end. We are able to observe some changes in interactions as well as some that continue as before. Sue has become more involved with the other members although Anne continues to speak only to Sue. Mary and John are now participating. Bill is still speaking to the group as a whole but why does no one respond to him?

Now, you might ask, "What do I do with these observations?" Well, you can base some of your future interventions on the process observed or you may want to use your observations as feedback to the members. Comments such as, "Bill, I notice that members don't often speak to you and I'm wondering if that might be because you never speak to any members directly?," or, "Anne, do you feel uncomfortable with the other members as I notice that you only talk to Sue?," can elicit important information about the members. Such questions also frequently serve as catalysts to involve the members in discussing the process in the group and the issues raised. By occasionally checking the group process through the use of interaction diagrams, the leader-therapist can compare her own perceptions of the interactive process with the pattern that appears on the diagram. For example, say interaction patterns are charted at different times to give two sample segments of a group. It can be seen from Figure 10-4 that during this period only half the members are involved. In such a case the leader-

Figure 10-4. Interaction confined to verbal members.

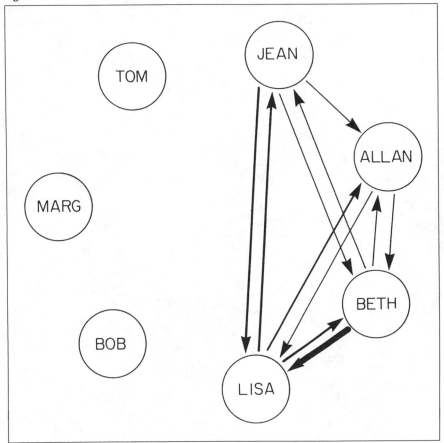

therapist may bring this to the attention of the members and suggest that a couple of the verbal members change seats with the quiet members. When verbal members are closely situated, their eye contact and interactions are likely to remain confined. If they are seated across from each other, then as they interact they are more likely to make some eye contact with others in the group, which will encourage the quiet members to participate. However, seating verbal members across from each other also has inherent problems. The two members, interacting only with each other across the group, tend to split the group, making it difficult for the members on either side to interact.

By putting Marg between Jean and Allan and moving Beth to Marg's position you intersperse the quiet members with the verbal members. In the next Figure 10-5, the expected interactions between the verbal members are shown by solid arrows. Because the quiet members are now more in the line of vision of the

Figure 10-5. Possible effects of relocating verbal members.

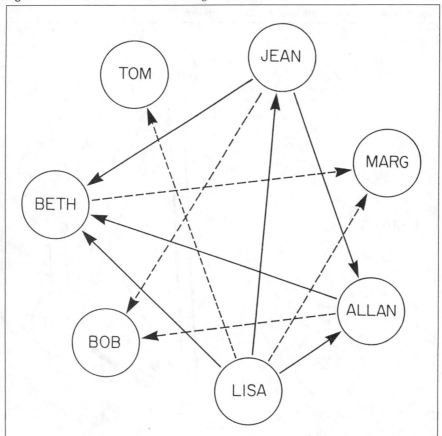

verbal members, they are more apt to receive eye contact, feel included, and respond. If Lisa now speaks to Beth or Jean as she did before, then Tom, being in between the two, is likely to feel less excluded and is more likely to try and get involved in the discussion as well.

To summarize, it is probable that you will employ different methods for observing and analyzing your group in its various phases. There are times when you will wish to focus primarily on the interactions and other times when you will be more interested in the content. These interests will be reflected in your selected method of observation and analysis for any given session.

SUMMARY

Finding yourself analyzing your own personal social groups can be a hazard of becoming professionally skilled in group analysis. Obtaining the skill, however, is a must for the effective leader-therapist. Analysis enables you to understand more clearly the process occurring in your group and forms the basis from which interventions or changes are made. However, even when skilled, much of what comes out of your analysis will be conjecture and should be checked out with the members, or over time, for accuracy. On the other hand, some observations do glean the quality of information that leads to obvious interpretation or conclusions.

Observing and analyzing your group is in some respects similar to doing a mental status examination. It is usual when first learning to do a mental status examination to employ headings as reminders of areas of focus such as sensorium, thought processes, memory, and behavior. In analyzing your group there are also certain areas which must be focused on and brought into your perpetual awareness. To assist you in this process you may want to use a form, check list, or survey sheet. Such aids will serve to remind you to look for and observe the quality and extent of verbal participation, nonverbal cues, member roles, subgroups, influence, and emotional tone. Later on you may feel that reminders are no longer necessary, but even when you reach the stage of skilled observer it can be useful to occasionally use some tool as an observation check.

CHAPTER 11

Goals and Norms

Before starting on a journey,
we first develop some idea of
the destination.
                    — JOHN BRILHART

Everything we do in life, be it sleeping, working, or playing, is goal-directed behavior. When we sleep we hope to be rested when we awake. For most people financial reward is a primary goal of work, although there are those who would say that enjoyment in work and a feeling of being productive is of more importance. Certainly enjoyment, fun, and pleasure are the basic goals of play.

Often we cannot achieve our goals alone, so we seek out others who can assist, are similarly involved, or who have the same goals. If we wish to become an occupational therapist we apply to programs in occupational therapy. If we wish to play baseball we join a baseball team. If we have a keen concern about acid rain we may try to find others who share this concern and move toward organizing a group to lobby the government for some specific actions. In each case we become part of a goal-directed group and in each case there exist goals that the group as a whole identifies and goals that members of the group identify for themselves as their own goals. These are known as *group goals* and *individual goals*. For example, the baseball team we join may have the goal of winning the pennant as their group goal whereas an individual player's goal might be to hit a home run. Examining the concept of goals, Palazzolo (1981) identifies individual needs and group needs as well as *individual goals* and *group goals*, but notes the difficulty in differentiating between them. He defines *individual needs* as "forces within the individual, the existence of which is inferred through behavior directed toward the achievement of a goal" (p. 22).

To carry on with the baseball example, the individual's need may be to gain recognition or approval for performance from his father. He sees hitting a home run as a possible means of achieving this, so he directs his efforts, perhaps through constant batting practice, toward this goal.

Table 11-1 gives examples of individual needs, the type of group through which the individual might meet the need, and what the related individual goal might be. This helps to clarify the differences between individual needs and individual goals.

Group needs, as defined by Palazzolo (1981) are "forces which develop out of group affiliation, and which promote concerted activity directed toward the achievement of a goal acceptable to the group as a whole" (p. 22).

Here is an example reflecting this definition: Members of a ward's recreational group become dissatisfied with the confinement and lack of variety in activities offered by the staff and propose ideas and methods for expanding or diversifying the recreational program.

On the other hand, Barker, Wahlers, Cegala, and Kibler (1979) believe that the same definition can be applied to both individual and group needs and their definition is that "a need is a perceived discrepancy between perception of present conditions or status and perception of what should be or what would be an ideal status" (p 39). Due to the difficulties in differentiating between individual and group needs the optimal situation is one where individual needs are similar enough, and blend sufficiently to become the needs realized by the group as a whole. Noting this to be the most favorable case, Palazzolo (1981) then points out the possibility of other less favorable situations occurring in the relationship between individual and group needs. These situations can occur when:

Table 11-1. RELATIONSHIP: NEEDS, GROUP CHOICE AND GOALS

Need	Group choice	Goal
Companionship	Friendship group	Friendship
Love and affection	Marital dyads Family groups	Sexual and emotional support
Achievement	Occupational groups	Recognition and promotion
Knowledge	Educational groups	Diploma, degree, honors
Public recognition	Political groups	Elected or appointed office
Competition	Athletic teams	Winning
Aggression	The military	Defeating the enemy, domination
Altruism	Social service groups Volunteer groups	Well-being of others, helping the underprivileged

Source: From C. S. Palazzolo (1981), *Small groups: An introduction* (p. 24). New York: Van Nostrand Reinhold.

a. The needs of individuals and those of the group are so incompatible that neither can be fulfilled.
b. The group may function in a way that realizes the group's needs but not those of the individual.
c. Some members may work only toward meeting their individual needs to the exclusion and detriment, if not the destruction, of the group as a whole.

Since needs, both group and individual, are seen as precursors to the establishment of goals, the above tenets apply equally to the blending and integration of individual and group goals. If the needs of the individual members of the group are similar and compatible they will integrate to become the group needs. In turn, these unified needs will facilitate and promote the group's successful functioning and attainment of its goals.

GOALS

Following from the discussion on needs, goals can be said to be the objectives established in order to satisfy needs. As defined by Barker, Wahlers, Cegala, and Kibler (1979) *"a goal is the objective or end result that a group or an individual seeks to achieve"* (p. 63). It is that which is valued sufficiently by an individual or a group to motivate action toward its achievement (Johnson & Johnson, 1982).

As noted earlier, there are two main types of goals: group and individual. The latter are also referred to as personal goals. Important to the success of the group is for the needs of individual members to be compatible with the needs of the group and it is equally important that the individual goals of members be congruent with the group goals. It should also be mentioned that both individuals and groups can and usually do have primary and secondary goals (Dunphy, 1972). Your stated primary goal in joining a bridge club may be a desire to learn to play bridge, with your secondary goal being to make new friends. For someone else these goals could be reversed, and they see the opportunity to join the club as an excellent opportunity to make new friends, with the learning to play bridge as secondary but also of value. If we follow along with this example to the actual bridge club meeting where the above two members are present, we get an idea of what can happen when individual goals are different, even though they are considered to be compatible. Let us say that you are the person whose primary goal is to learn to play bridge. During the play you are concentrating on trying to remember the rules, bids, and cards played. However, your partner or one of the opposing players, who joined the club to make new friends, keeps up a steady stream of personal questions as a way of getting to know you (or another player) better with the hopes of starting a new friendship. The problems, quick to arise in such a situation, are obvious. You, and probably the remaining two players, will have difficulty concentrating, forget the bids made or which cards have been played, and are likely to become annoyed by all the questions and chatter. So the player whose goal was to make friends has instead irritated those present and as a result has possibly lost the opportunity or chance of obtaining his goal. Although a bridge foursome is a highly structured group with inherent rules and procedures, the same kind of conflicts and problems can arise in less structured groups where members have considerably different goals.

In discussing the relationship between individual and group goals, Zander, Natsoulas, and Thomas (1978) present four distinct but closely related concepts regarding goals. The first, a *member's goal for the group,* is an end result toward which a member tries to influence group movement. In therapy groups this member's goal is frequently the same as the leader-therapist's goal. For example, the leader-therapist of an assertiveness group may have in mind the degree of confidence and independence that it is realistic to expect from the members and may exert pressure on the group to work toward this level of achievement. Secondly, the *group goal* "is a region of positive valence toward which a group tends to locomote and is usually some synthesis of the members' goals for the group" (p. 168). To continue our example of the assertiveness group, the group goal might be for members to become more independent and assertive and thus be better able to deal with their individual problems. Next is the *group's goal for a member,* which can involve pressure being exerted by the group on a member from a you-can-do-it position. The pressure, which can be slight or intense, may be for the member to try harder, to risk more, to achieve a certain level, or just to become more involved. Lastly is the *personal goal,* which is the private goal that each individual sets for himself in keeping with his needs, aspirations, strengths, and weaknesses as he sees them. A personal goal of a member of an assertiveness group might be to learn how to interact with his father in a way that is not antagonistic and allows him to get his point of view across.

The four types of goals are interrelated and a change in any one of them will affect the others to some degree. Zander, Natsoulas, and Thomas (1978) describe this as "a circular causal relationship among these four goals," which occurs in the direction in which they have been presented. This means that if the *member's* (or leader-therapist's) *goal* for the group changes, this will affect all the remaining goals in sequence. It can be seen that this interrelatedness of goals has ramifications not only for group and individual success but also in the selection and referral of clients to specific groups.

GOALS IN THERAPY GROUPS

In most social or working groups you have individual goals, group goals, and tasks. Tasks are performed in order to accomplish the group's goals (Barker, Wahlers, Cegala, & Kibler, 1983). In task-oriented therapy groups the task is often only the medium around which the most important aspects of the group occur. It is true that tasks are carried out in order to accomplish goals, but in some instances they are not of great import in and of themselves. In these cases the important things are the interactions, behaviors, feelings, roles, in fact everything that occurs in the group in the process of doing the task. Completion of the task may not be of paramount importance. More will be said about this in Chapter 13. Establishing goals in therapy groups is an important aspect of the group but can be a difficult process. Many clients are not practiced or skilled in consciously defining goals in their everyday lives. They tend to proceed with work and play and generally living their life, but if they were to be asked, "What are your goals at this moment in your life?," they would more than likely be hard pressed to give a definite answer.

This lack of goals can, in fact, be part of the underlying problems that clients are experiencing: they have no clear, formulated goals to give their life meaning. Possible responses to the question might go something like these: "To do a good job" . . . "To have a good time" . . . "To enjoy life." Similarly, vague, generalized goals are produced by clients in therapy groups. Initially, if a client is asked to state his goals for being in the group a probable answer would be, "To get better," or even, "I don't know. My doctor [therapist] just told me to come to the group." As well, there are those clients who only see their goal in the group as a means of obtaining discharge ("If I come to the group I think I'll get discharged faster"). Still others come to the group to be "done to" and their response goes something like this: "I'm going to get therapy [treatment] here." And so it falls to the leader-therapist to be facilitative in helping group members to, first, learn how to define goals, and then to define goals that are meaningful and appropriate for them as individuals. These goals must be in keeping with the overall goals of the group which are frequently established by the leader-therapist.

LEADER-THERAPIST GOALS

Groups in occupational therapy most often have a theme which globally reflects the nature of the group and, by deduction, the nature of the goals of the group.

A life skills group is going to have, as an overall goal, one of helping members become more functional in coping with the demands and exigencies of day-to-day living. A self-awareness group will be focused on increasing members' awareness of their own needs, feelings, attitudes, and behaviors. Clients are usually referred to such groups following an initial assessment by an occupational therapist, the treatment team as a whole, or as happens in some settings, by individually specified team members. Results of the assessment should determine areas of both competence and difficulty for the client. Based on these strengths and weaknesses, and in consultation and discussion with the client, the therapist will select the types of groups felt to be most beneficial for the client. This is the stage at which the client, together with the therapist, begins to establish his goals. The goals established at this time may be several and more global than specific. For example, "lack of self-confidence" may have been found to be a problem for the client as determined by the assessment process. The therapist suggests and explains to the client how an assertiveness training group could be useful in helping the client develop more self-confidence and so it is agreed that the client will attend the group.

As mentioned earlier, it is the role of the leader-therapist to facilitate and assist in the definition of goals by group members. In doing so the leader-therapist must always keep in mind that the individual goals defined by each member of the group must be compatible with those defined by the other members and also with those of the group as a whole: the group goals. The latter are where the leader-therapist's goals for the group are usually most apparent. In the example of an assertiveness training group the leader-therapist may have determined through past experience which assertive techniques can be most useful and most easily learned. Her goals may include ways of structuring the group to ensure opportunities for group members to experience and learn these techniques. She must make sure, however, that these techniques will help the members progress toward achieving their individual goals.

INDIVIDUAL GOALS

When a new member joins a group, especially if the setting is in a hospital, it is most likely to be a group that is ongoing and has been functioning for some time. Outpatient programs or community clinics are more apt to run groups in a series of sessions, more like a course, and prospective members are then required to wait until the next course starts. In this case, where the first session is the beginning of the group for all, it is logical to use the first meeting or part of it as a time for members, in discussion with the leader-therapist and other members, to establish their individual goals for the sessions. However, in an ongoing group this opportunity for goal setting is not as available and can too easily be overlooked. It is frequently the case that the new member arrives, is welcomed to the group, introductions are made, the activities of the group are explained, and the group begins. The wise leader-therapist will take a little time at the outset to facilitate not only the integration of the new member but initiate the process of goal setting by the new member. The following ideas can work together:

1. Suggest that group members share one or more of their individual goals
with the newcomer. This actually can be of benefit to the ongoing members as
well as the new member. To state or restate their goals like this can be very helpful to present members by giving them the opportunity to clarify and recon-
firm their own goals.
2. Members could be invited to share one thing they have learned from the
sessions they have participated in. This too can be very beneficial to ongoing
members. Directed to think about it, some members will be surprised to realize
just what they have (or have not) learned.
3. Ask the new member to "tell us a little bit about yourself" and "do you have
any thoughts on what you would like to achieve or get out of this group?"
4. If the new member appears quite tense and ill at ease, it might be wiser to
begin the group after introductions, suggesting that the new member might like
to "see what goes on here." Later on in the session the new member can be encouraged to explore his problems, needs, and areas of difficulty. From and by
these interactions, he can be helped in defining goals to work toward while in
the group.

Follow-up

It is important that time is taken periodically in a group session to evaluate the
progress that members are making toward the achievement of their individual
goals. This can be accomplished by (1) the members sharing their own assessment of their progress; (2) by members giving each other feedback, and (3) by
the leader-therapist giving members feedback. At this point members may also
wish to formulate some additional goals based on what they have experienced
and learned from the group so far.
   Some goals are very immediate and visible. For example, a very shy person
may have as a goal that he will speak up voluntarily at least twice in each session. When the goal is this obvious it is easy for success to be observed, which
in turn makes it easy for other members to give encouraging feedback. Other
goals are frequently abstract, although the more that members can be urged to
make their goals specific in terms of observable behavior the easier it is for
them to experience a sense of achievement (Palazzolo, 1981). This is where the
leader-therapist and other group members can be helpful. If a member (in an
assertiveness training group) says, "I want to be able to stand up for myself
more," he can be encouraged to explore with the other members the ways in
which he would behave if he were to "stand up for himself more." This might
draw comments like, "I would say what I want," "I'd say no (or yes) more
often," or, "I'd give my opinion." These are observable behaviors that can be
counted and as such make better goals than the general statement of standing
up for oneself. They are better because the behavior can be recognized by the
individual, the group members, staff, and other clients, so the chances of receiving feedback are greater.
   It should be understood that clients are to work on their goals both in and out
of the group so a follow-up discussion would deal with both situations. The

member's own report might be that on a certain occasion he was able to say that he did not like the music being played so loud in the lounge. Feedback from group members might be that he was contributing his ideas more often during lunch conversation, and feedback from the leader-therapist might indicate pleasure that the member was now more able to suggest or ask for things in group, like role-playing a specific situation.

GOALS VIS-À-VIS TASKS

Most groups that are run by occupational therapists involve a task of some nature. A task may be defined as "an act, or its result, that a small group is required, either by itself or someone else, to perform" (Barker, Wahlers, Cegala, & Kibler, 1983, p. 41). Tasks differ widely from group to group. They vary from role-playing life situations, to solving puzzles, writing down what you like or do not like about something, reaching a consensus, or making up a monthly budget. Sometimes these tasks are confused with the goals of the group. In a consensus task, although the purpose may be to reach agreement on the correct order of the information, the goals for the group are varied: to work together cooperatively, to enable members to experience both leading and following while becoming aware of their style of participation, to allow members to experience both success and frustration, to see how the group makes decisions, and for the group, to assume and deal with the responsibility of completing the task. This last may or may not occur and depending on the goals of the group may or may not be important.

Another task could have real meaning for the group in and of itself and in such an instance differentiating between task and goal may be irrelevant. The overall goal of a cooking group may be to organize, prepare, and serve a meal. Accomplishing this goal will require many tasks: deciding on the menu, making up a shopping list, doing the shopping, dividing up preparation responsibilities, cooking, and serving the meal. These tasks are performed in order to achieve the overall goal, but they also have inherent goals. For example, in drawing up a menu the inherent goal is to formulate a menu that is balanced and includes all the appropriate items.

The most important issue around the relationship between goals and tasks is for the leader-therapist to be conscious of both at all times. Every group leader hopes that the group will embrace the task enthusiastically and that all members will become involved and work toward its completion. With certain tasks, though, it is all too easy for the leader-therapist to become involved with the task to the point of forgetting about the goals of individual members and even the overall purpose of the group. Frequently the leader-therapist will participate in the task as a means of modeling and to minimize the leadership role. In such instances it is critical that the leader-therapist achieve a balance between observing and facilitating the group process, and participating in the task. Even after extensive experience in leading groups there are times when the task, the discussion, or certain members will captivate the leader's interest so completely that she becomes a group member totally and all leadership roles are disregarded.

A word of caution is in order. Groups are powerful vehicles for therapy, which is why they are used so extensively as a treatment modality. The sharing and intimacy experienced in groups paves the way for closeness and caring to develop among the members. The leader-therapist herself will experience varying degrees of closeness with different members and in different groups. She must always be aware of and monitor these feelings, making sure she does not cross the invisible line and use the group for her own personal therapy.

HIDDEN AGENDAS

Whenever individuals come together to interact, the interaction occurs on two levels. On one level the interaction is conscious and its purpose is usually publicly stated. This purpose can be to accomplish a task, reach an objective, or to work on problems, and this is considered to be the public or surface agenda (Napier & Gershenfeld, 1973). But under this public knowledge of purpose are "the conflicting motives, desires, aspirations and emotional reactions held by the group members" (Bradford, 1978b, p. 85). These covert needs and desires of the members are called *hidden agendas.*

INDIVIDUAL HIDDEN AGENDAS

Hidden agendas held by individuals may be conscious or unconscious and either way they can affect the overall functioning of the group (Sampson & Marthas, 1981). It is this influence that should be recognized when considering hidden agendas and not whether they are good or bad. Bradford (1978b) notes that a good time to observe hidden agendas is during the initial stage of a group. To deal with the tensions that are present at the beginning of a group, members tend to behave self-protectively while making advances toward other members in keeping with their own needs and desires. If allowed to take its course this process of probing and exploring by group members can be constructive in the dispersion of hidden agendas. In a therapy group a member who has a strong aversion to all persons in authority, may test the leader to discover the degree of imposed authority, or as a protection he may try to wrest the position of authority from the leader-therapist. For example, he may ask the leader about a ward rule that he knows has just been changed. This outward behavior appears straightforward and may even convey a message of wanting to be a "good client" by knowing and following the rules. However, when the leader-therapist responds with the old rule the member corrects her, thus challenging her position as authority figure. The leader-therapist who recognizes this maneuver for what it is can, by conciliatory interaction with the member and the group, diffuse the attack while retaining her leadership role intact. A less experienced leader-therapist may feel threatened, react defensively, and find herself in a heated dispute with the member.

An example of a less hostile hidden agenda is when a member attends the group only to receive "Brownie points" for personal gain, such as a weekend pass. Another personal reason a member might harbor is to use the group as a forum for displaying behaviors to impress or catch the interest of a particular fellow client, perhaps a member of the opposite sex. These members, not committed to or interested in the purpose or value of the group, can be distracting and disruptive to the overall process and to the efforts of the other members.

GROUP HIDDEN AGENDAS

The group as a whole can also have hidden agendas. For example, if the group does not like the assigned task, their hidden agenda may be one of sabotage. While this intent is never verbalized members accept and even encourage undermining behaviors such as lack of cooperation, lack of participation, disruptive participation, or apathy. Another group may be resistant to disclosing feelings or engaging in personal sharing. In this case the group can defend against expectations of such interactions by sticking to superficial dialogue, joking, laughing, or going off the topic deliberately. In this way a group's hidden agenda can control the interactions and become established as an informal or implicit norm for the group. Directly challenging a member or the group about harboring a hidden agenda is not likely to be productive (Sampson & Marthas, 1981). If the members who were constantly joking and laughing were asked if they were doing so to avoid intimacy, they are highly unlikely to answer yes. Rather, the leader-therapist on examining her interpretation of their behavior, might ask herself, "What does it mean?" "Are the members feeling pushed?" "Are the expectations for sharing too high?" "Is the process moving too fast for their comfort?" Based on hypothetical answers to these questions the leader-therapist may make modifications in leadership tactics, tasks, and style.

LEADER-THERAPIST HIDDEN AGENDAS

The leader-therapist may also have conscious or unconscious hidden agendas. On a conscious level the leader-therapist may plan a group in a specific way in order to facilitate desired behaviors in the group. The plan might be to select a task that requires each group member to participate frequently if the task is to be completed. In choosing this particular activity the leader-therapist is planning around one member of the group — the silent member. Her idea is that through the use of this task the silent member will have to become involved in the group but can do so through a nonthreatening natural process.

On an unconscious level the hidden agenda of the leader-therapist may be "that of maintaining his leadership at any cost. The position of influence and power is pleasing, and he will not relinquish it" (Bradford, 1978b, p. 91). In another instance the leader-therapist may enforce her leadership role because she fears "what might happen" if she were to lose control of the group. This fear may be unfounded in terms of the group members' behaviors, but because it is beneath her awareness, perhaps (in psychoanalytic terms) stemming from unresolved childhood issues of control, it continues to influence her leadership style. Behaviors displayed by a leader-therapist to maintain her power and control could be: disregarding ideas and suggestions from members, disagreeing with members, invoking rules, and using sarcasm. On recognition of any of these behaviors in herself, the leader-therapist must try to analyze her feelings as objectively as possible and attempt to alter or modify her manner.

NORMS

All groups, social and therapeutic, formal and informal, have sets of standards that govern the way in which members' behaviors are judged. These standards are known as *norms*. Norms also "specify the kinds of behaviors that are expected of group members" (Hare, 1976, p. 24). A behavior cannot be described as being intrinsically conforming or deviant. A behavior can only be deviant or conforming in relationship to the norms of the group within which it occurs (Hare, 1976). A man who swears while sharing the bench with his fellow team players at a football game may not be considered deviant. He may be conforming to the way his team members express their frustrations and disappointments throughout the game. Given other settings, for example, with family or friends, this same man may express his frustrations without profanity. He is accepting and abiding by the social norms that he feels are present in the two different situations.

According to Palazzolo (1981), "Group norms define the limits within which behavior is deemed acceptable or appropriate" (p. 28). The acceptance by individuals of being controlled by norms or adhering to norms is part of the socialization process that occurs as one experiences society as a whole. This learning is then extended to specific and smaller units of society. Individuals come to believe that conforming to the norms of the group is what is best for them and best for the group. If individuals are accepted as having a basic need to *belong* (Maslow, 1962), then this need becomes a strong motivator for them to behave in ways that will ensure their acceptability in any given group. By doing this they are accepting the norms of the group. Each group to which a person belongs will have different norms and each group will enforce adherence to these norms in different ways. Some groups will tolerate deviance from a particular norm or norms by certain individuals, whereas other groups require strict conformity.

Norms function as the rules of the game and assist in the smooth running of a group or unit. They are guidelines of behavior within which members can behave with some degree of confidence. Nixon (1979) speaks of norms as being *shared expectations*. By this he means they are not individual expectations, but standards that group members "collectively hold and apply to each other" (p. 110). The application of norms may vary depending on the status of the individual. By virtue of her role the leader-therapist may be exempt from certain norms or a valued member may flaunt nonconforming behavior, but because of the person's value to the group the behavior may be tolerated. This is not to say the behavior will necessarily be tolerated forever.

The group may eventually realize that normative behavior is of more importance to the group than the value of the member, at which point pressure may be applied to the member to conform or to leave. Norms touch on all aspects of our lives — how we express feelings, how we eat, and so on. Children internalize the behavior of parents and take on these behaviors as their own. Even the roles of parenting are internalized by children, which is why children who have been abused frequently grow up to become abusive parents. These are the norms they have been socialized to, and hence are those they have adopted.

Every family is a unique social system and as such has its own norms and standards of behavior. A family member who behaves in a way that is in conflict with or outside the accepted standards of that family is seen as being deviant and may be ostracized. Monane (1967) says, "Psychological disturbance in one member of a family . . . carries a profound impact on other family members and upon the family as a system" (pp. 23–24). Some families have such a high investment in presenting an image of the perfect family that they ignore or cover for a troubled member rather than mar the family image by seeking help. What they are doing in this instance is elevating the norm of "we don't have any problems" to the highest level of importance.

EXPLICIT NORMS

Norms can be divided into two categories: *explicit* and *implicit,* or *formal* and *informal* (Hare, 1976). Explicit or formal norms are standards or guidelines that are clearly stated and of which all members are aware. Information concerning formal norms may be given to all new members as they join the group (e.g., "Smoking is not allowed during group sessions" . . . "No one is allowed to go out for coffee once the session has started"). Such explicit norms are usually formally established for the betterment of the group as a whole. They may be decided on by the group as a whole or by the leader alone. Frequently a norm established by the leader, such as, "All members must come to group on time," is embraced by the group members as they come to realize the disruptive results of members arriving late.

IMPLICIT NORMS

Implicit or informal norms are not formally stated but evolve from prior standards or behaviors brought by members to the group and which the members as a unit embrace. It is more difficult for an observer to ascertain what implicit norms are operating in a group than it is to discover the explicit norms. A woman once moved with her lieutenant-commander husband to a naval base. Initially she occasionally invited the neighbors' wives to her home for coffee. Over the course of a few weeks she was aware that not one neighbor had reciprocated with an invitation to her home for coffee. Hurt by this she confided to her husband that the neighbor women must not like her. His response, "Well, of course they won't invite you because their husbands are lieutenants," quite shocked her. He pursued the issue by asking if she ever considered inviting the commander's wife for coffee and she promptly replied, "No, of course not." At this point she realized that for certain forms of socializing the unwritten rule or protocol of the military base was to invite only colleagues of equal or lesser status. More obvious perhaps, as an example of an implicit norm, is the bank manager who "knows" it is inappropriate for him to go to his office in blue jeans and a sweatshirt.

Implicit norms can cause intense pressure. The pressure comes from feeling impelled to be and act like others in the hopes of being accepted. Such norms are evident and especially strong throughout the adolescent and teenage years. All parents have experienced the protestation, "No one wears those!," or, "No one does that!," in response to efforts to convince an adolescent to wear certain clothing or do certain things. The power and control of such norms should not be underestimated. A bright 16-year-old girl was drawn to a school group who were nonachievers, but as demonstrated by their laughter and high jinks they appeared to have a great deal of fun. Because of her good marks they resisted her overtures of friendliness with taunts of "teacher's pet." Six months later, when she was failing three of her courses, she was grudgingly given acceptance by the group.

In therapeutic groups explicitly stated norms might be, "members must attend group," or, "members must arrive on time." Another could be that neither smoking nor eating is allowed while in group. Implicit norms are likely to vary from one therapeutic group to another and are more difficult to discern. In one group the norm may be for members to share feelings openly including negative reactions to others, whereas in another group the norm may be to share feelings and reactions, but only if they are positive. The extent of conformity among members to the norm of sharing is often directly related to the level of cohesiveness in the group and this norm may change as the group progresses.

Generally, norms cannot be considered to be good or bad. It is the effect they have on the group that is evaluated. Members may see the group as a place to vent the frustrations they feel about the treatment regimen or the ward schedule and at certain times this may be appropriate and constructive. However, if the griping continues and a norm, "the group is the place to complain," is established, then other personal and more productive issues may be excluded or banned.

REACTING TO NORMS

Four options are open to a group member from which he may choose his way of handling an established group norm (Hare, 1976). If he agrees with and feels positively about the norm he is likely to conform and even strengthen the norm. Should he disagree with the norm, believing it to be a poor standard for himself or the group, he can try to convince the other group members that the norm should be changed. If these attempts fail, or if he decides against trying to make changes, he has the option to ignore the norm and behave as he wishes.

Ignoring an established norm of the group moves the individual into the role of a deviant. A more definitive reaction, if he finds he cannot abide by the standard, would be for him to leave the group. Summarizing, the four options are:

1. Conform to the norm.
2. Try to change the norm.
3. Remain deviant.
4. Leave the group.

The most successful way of changing established norms is through discussion. Frequently members are not aware that implicit norms are operating in the group. A norm might be established that when a particular person speaks, no matter what he says, the rest of the group argues with him. Members may demonstrate surprise, and perhaps some defensiveness, or disagreement when it is pointed out to them that they are behaving in this manner. The ensuing discussion will more than likely have a moderating affect on this particular behavior. It could also have an effect on the member with whom they constantly argue. Perhaps he is also unaware that certain of his behaviors, like always thinking he is right, provoke others to argument. There are also occasions when merely making an observation of conforming behavior is sufficient to bring about change. Reactions of, "I thought we were supposed to do . . .," or, "How is it that everyone . . .," will frequently lead to dissolution of unproductive norms or behaviors.

By role modeling and encouraging desired behavior the leader-therapist can impact on the norms of the group. For example, if she confronts a member who uses profane language with, "John, I don't like it when you swear," this gives a message to the members that swearing is not O.K., at least not O.K. with the leader. By doing this she is not stating an explicit norm ("There will be no swearing in the group"), but rather she is submitting an opinion on a specific behavior in hopes of preventing the behavior from becoming an accepted standard. In a therapeutic setting group members often see the leader-therapist as the authority and thus, "what she says, goes." In this way the leader-therapist can be instrumental in establishing norms. To carry the above example further, at a later group session where a new member does use swearwords it is quite likely that he will be informed by another member that "swearing isn't allowed here." At this stage the norm has become more of an explicit norm.

The leader-therapist can role-model in less directive ways that can also impact on the norms of a group. By being open and sharing with her feelings, both positive and negative, she conveys the message that such behavior is acceptable. In many groups, especially newly formed ones, the norm of making only positive comments to one another is easily established. When a member does or says something that is visibly upsetting to the others, another norm may be to say nothing, but to ignore the member who has caused the reaction. In this instance, the leader can share how she feels about what the member said or did and ask others how they felt. This intervention may open the door for more honest reactions and expand the norm to the sharing of both positive and negative feelings.

The leader-therapist needs to closely observe and analyze the process in her group to reach an awareness of the norms that are in effect. If she feels they are inhibiting group progress, she should try to facilitate movement toward their dissolution. If the norms are felt to be positive and productive in nature, she will want to be reinforcing. Of most importance, though, is the awareness. Knowing what norms are operating contributes to the leader-therapist's understanding of the behaviors and actions of the group members.

SUMMARY

People are drawn to groups for various reasons, one of which is that they discern the group as a place where they can respond to a felt need and act on it through the goals of the group. For example, people who have strong spiritual needs will be attracted to others who share their needs and by joining together they can delineate goals that will find avenues of expression based on these needs. Unfortunately, not all persons are able to recognize their needs, and even if they are, not all are able to satisfy them through goal setting. This is especially true of persons who are experiencing emotional problems. Because of this it frequently falls to the leader-therapist to assist the members of her group in recognizing their needs and, based on this knowledge, assist them in formulating appropriate goals.

The goals of some groups are obvious from the assigned designation, such as a life skills group. However, before clients are referred to a designated group, their needs must be assessed by a therapist or the team and a determination made that these needs may be met in this particular group. In other groups the goals are specifically formulated from the needs of the assembled members. Whichever is the case the group must be planned so that the goals will promote therapeutic outcomes for the members. To do this, the mix of individual and group needs and individual and group goals must blend, and success comes from finding a compatible mix.

Success can also depend on the presence or absence of hidden agendas and the norms that are operating in the group. The latter fall into two categories, explicit and implicit, with the implicit being those that usually evolve within the group and can affect the process in either a positive or a negative way. Explicit norms are usually stated at the beginning of the group or as required or appropriate. It is important for the leader-therapist to give consideration to hidden agendas and norms whenever she is observing or analyzing the process in a group.

CHAPTER 12

Membership

We're all in this together —
by ourselves.
                    — LILY TOMLIN

A therapeutic group differs from social groups. Indeed, its purpose is to be "therapeutic." This term is defined in the *New Lexicon Webster's Dictionary* (1987) as meaning "curative." *Funk and Wagnalls Standard College Dictionary* (1982) adds, "having healing qualities." The former definition is emphasized in Yalom's (1970) "curative factors" presented in Chapter 1. We would not expect a social group to be "curative." Rather we would expect it to be enjoyable, fun, and perhaps informative. Taking the broadest sense of the word, though, we might join a social group, or perhaps a book club, as a means of "curing" our loneliness and in this sense the group could be said to be therapeutic. However, the main goal of most book clubs is a literary one, accomplished through presentations and discussions on books, not one of curing the loneliness of its members. In a therapeutic group the main goal is for the experience to remedy or alleviate members' problems — in effect, to have a curative effect. The initial formation of any group requires careful planning and thoughtful answers to some basic questions. In addition to answering those outlined in Figure 12-1, the leader-therapist needs to consider some other factors such as, "What will the members do?" . . . "How long will the sessions last?" . . . "How big will the group be?" . . . "Are there enough members?" . . . "Are there too many members?," and so on. All are critical issues. Questions of size and composition along with membership roles are addressed in this chapter.

SIZE

Size is an important consideration when forming any type of group. The optimal number of members for a therapy group is thought to be five or six (Levine, 1979), although Yalom (1983) states that six to 10 is the number of members preferred by most clinicians. It is important that every member have an opportunity to participate and there is evidence to suggest that to achieve "mutual

Figure 12-1. Pregroup issue. (Source: Adapted from C. L. Kell and P. R. Corts, *Fundamentals of Effective Group Communication.* New York: Macmillan, 1980.)

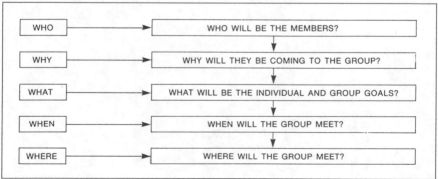

responsivity" in a discussion group, fewer than eight to 10 persons should be involved (Steiner, 1972). In their observations of five free discussion groups over 3 to 4 years, Zimet and Schneider (1969) found that not only did verbal interaction decrease as the size of the group increased but that the interactions also became less personal. Investigations by Castore (1962) indicated a marked decrease in member-to-member interactions when the size of the group reached nine persons. While Levine believes that four is the minimum number for a group, Yalom suggests that even a group of three can occasionally function very successfully. Most importantly, the appropriate number of members for any given group will depend on the purpose, structure, and capacities of the individuals involved (Levine, 1979). Wide fluctuations in size are usually unavoidable and the number of persons available for a group often depends on admissions and discharges, events on the ward or unit, and the therapeutic requirements of the clients.

The size of the group will determine the extent to which interpersonal relationships and hence cohesiveness will develop among the members. Ten or more members may function productively in client self-government groups, social groups, or counseling groups, but one would not expect any depth of intimacy to develop in these groups (Geller, 1982; Napier & Gershenfeld, 1973). While Sampson and Marthas (1981) point out the increase in number and variety of resources in a larger membership, they also note the correlation between an increase in group size and a decrease in time for member participation. Perhaps the latter is why Luft (1984) says that, "morale tends to be lower in larger groups than in comparable smaller ones" (p. 23).

An ongoing group can survive periodic low membership sessions since some degree of unity will have already been established. This may, however, result in the nature of the group changing due to the missing roles of the absent members. It is important that the leader-therapist expect and be sensitive to differences and changes in the group when members leave the group, are away, or new members join. When such incidents occur, as mentioned earlier under termination, the leader-therapist must be facilitative in helping the members adapt to the changes in the group climate (Loomis, 1979).

COMPOSITION

Membership of therapy groups is determined in a variety of ways. On a ward or unit where the team approach is used, the clients on each team may be included in a psychotherapy group led by staff from their particular team. A different strategy is to relegate clients according to their level of functioning to selective groups: Low-functioning clients would meet together in one group while higher-functioning clients would gather together in a different group (Yalom, 1983). Membership in task groups usually depends on identified problems, level of functioning, and the projected goals of the clients.

Whether the reference is to diagnosis, age, sex, or the underlying psychopathologic condition, there are discrepant views on the issue of homogeneity or heterogeneity of membership in groups (Berne, 1966; Furst, 1975). It has been suggested that members who share similar demographics such as age, sex, education, and economic status, but who differ, for example, in degree of extroversion, humor, talkativeness, shyness, and compliance, are likely to function well together (Bertcher & Maple, 1977). Donohue (1982) makes a case for the "identification group," a group where membership is based on same age and sex. An identification group, she believes, gives members a feeling of "solidarity" that leaves them "with a feeling of relative comfort and security" (p. 5). Having had this positive experience, clients may be motivated to seek out a similar reference group as a means of support following discharge.

Homogeneous groups are believed by Hansen, Warner, and Smith (1976) to operate at a more superficial level and to be less successful in changing permanent behavior. However, these same authors credit homogeneous groups with being more cohesive, having better attendance, fewer conflicts, and faster relief of symptoms, and evidence of mutual support. Although Levine (1979) cautions that clients with severe depression are best treated in a group composed entirely of depressives, this author does not believe that this holds true for task or activity groups. Sadock and Kaplan (1972) promote heterogeneous groups for several reasons. They believe having men and women interact together in the same group offers more options for discussion and presents a more normative situation. They also point out that drawing members from only one category of illness or age level limits the group's resources by restricting its access to a variety of behavioral patterns and ways of functioning. Bennis and Shepard (1978) support this view by noting that in a heterogeneous group younger members can learn from older members and vice versa, disruptive members can benefit from feedback concerning their inappropriate behavior, and those who are withdrawn can be drawn out by more active members.

R. C. Erickson (1986) argues that, given the constraints of the setting, heterogeneous groups may be the only option open to leader-therapists on a short-stay inpatient unit. In this setting he suggests the issue is not assigning clients to groups according to their needs, but rather adjusting the goals of the current groups to meet the needs of the members. Toothman (1978) suggests that while it may be best to exclude persons who are acutely psychotic, extremely hostile and aggressive, very impulsive, or those with offensive mannerisms, he does recommend that membership should be representative of the general population. He also cautions that in all instances the selection or acceptance of members should reflect what the leader is able to tolerate or cope with. The reality of most situations is that the selection of members for any group is limited to the clients available and is influenced by their needs.

While occupational therapists may serve as leader-therapists in ward or unit groups, they more often select clients with similar problems or needs to meet in separate groups. To be most effective, occupational therapists should plan and organize their task groups in response to the needs of their current client population. For example, if a therapist has several clients who have become dysfunctional through withdrawal and dependence, she may establish a life skills group. Similarly, she might choose some of these same clients along with other more diffident clients to form a group in assertiveness training. In other settings the department of occupational therapy offers an assortment of task groups on an ongoing basis to which clients are referred as their problems and needs are determined. Another option for a department is to offer a basic group with various tasks to serve as an assessment. On admission, all clients initially attend this group so that the therapist(s) can determine the clients' needs and then refer them to the appropriate theme groups. Mosey (1970) formalized five levels of developmental groups, *parallel, project, egocentric-cooperative, cooperative,* and *mature,* specifically for clients who functioned below the expected level for participation in more interactive groups. Since a thorough presentation of these developmental groups can be found elsewhere, they will not be discussed here.

ROLES

Throughout any group session each individual member functions in one or more roles, and these may change as the group progresses. It is important for the leader-therapist to have an understanding of the various roles carried out by group members in order to grasp the overall dynamics of the group as they unfold. One way to do this is to look at the behaviors and interactions of individual members. This will enable you to determine the kinds of roles that each member assumes in the group and the role in which they primarily function. Determining these roles gives you important information about each member and how they interact with others. This does not necessarily mean they always behave in this role or manner outside of the group, but it is usually a good indicator of how they sometimes behave in their real-life groups such as family, work, or leisure. Becoming aware of the various roles that members assume not only helps you in understanding the group process but enables you to be therapeutic by increasing members' awareness of their behaviors and the inherent ramifications. Say you have a member who appears quite involved in the group, speaks up frequently, and seems quite interested in the other members. Overall he is considered to be a "good participator." However, on closer observation of this member's input you find that his interactions always have him in the role of questioner. Since this mode of interacting can be seen as a very effective way to keep the other members from getting to know him, it is important to determine what prompts him to keep the other members at a distance. By verbally making this observation (and the interpretation, if thought to be appropriate) to the member, you can facilitate a discussion of this aspect of the member's participation in the group — and perhaps in his life in general.

Several authors have presented methods for the analysis of group interaction (Bales, 1970) and functional member roles (Benne & Sheats, 1948; Dimock, 1985a). The classic functional member roles as laid down by Benne and Sheats (1948) have been utilized by many leaders, including this author. They are useful to the group observer in determining the manner of participation of the various group members. Because members usually confine themselves to a "limited range of roles" (Heap, 1977), the observer is able to formulate a defined image of each member's unique style of participation. As feedback to the members this information can be useful in helping members become more flexible by changing or expanding their roles. The leader-therapist must also be aware of her own assumption of these roles and through objective analysis or feedback from others define her own style. From this analysis she too may see a need for more flexibility or more definitive changes.

The member roles are classified into three general categories: (1) group task roles, (2) group building and maintenance roles, and (3) individual roles.

GROUP TASK ROLES

Group task roles are those that aid the group in defining and carrying out the task or goals of the group. These twelve roles may be seen as the working roles of the group.

1. The *initiator-contributor* suggests or proposes new ideas to the group. These may take the form of new goals, suggested solutions of difficulties encountered by the group, or different ways of regarding the group problem. The initiator-contributor can also be regarded as the person who mobilizes the group through his contribution, either initially or when the group gets bogged down.

2. The *information seeker* seeks clarification of offered suggestions in terms of their factual certainty and looks for authoritative information and facts pertinent to the problem at hand.

3. The *opinion seeker* does not focus primarily on the facts of the case but asks for clarification of the values relevant to the group's undertaking or of those involved in suggestions made.

4. The *information giver* offers facts or pieces of information which are "authoritative," or relates his own experience relevant to the group issue.

5. The *opinion giver* states his beliefs or opinions concerning any suggestions made. He emphasizes his proposal of what should become the group's view of pertinent values, rather than the relevant facts of information.

6. The *elaborator* explains suggestions in terms of examples or expanded meanings, offers a rationale for suggestions previously made, and speculates on how an idea or suggestion would work out if adopted by the group.

7. The *coordinator* tries to clarify the relationships between various ideas and suggestions, attempts to pull ideas and suggestions together, and tries to coordinate the activities of the various members or subgroups.

8. The *orienter* summarizes what has occurred and then defines the progress of the group, points to departures from agreed-upon aims or goals, and questions the direction of the group discussion.

9. The *evaluator-critic* assesses the accomplishments of the group in relation to some standard or set of standards that are relevant to the group task. Thus he may evaluate or question the "practicality," the "logic," or the "facts" of suggestions or of the manner of proceeding.

10. The *energizer* prods the group to action or decision, and attempts to stimulate or arouse the group to "greater" or "higher quality" activity.

11. The *procedural technician* is the handyman of the group and expedites group movement by performing routine tasks, for example, distributing materials, sharpening pencils, running audio-visuals, or rearranging the seating.

12. The *recorder* takes notes, makes lists, writes down suggestions, records group decisions, and generally serves as the "group memory."

GROUP BUILDING AND MAINTENANCE ROLES

Group members functioning in these roles are caring and oriented toward helping the group work well together. Their purpose is to build and maintain group-centered attitudes, behaviors, and activities. There are seven of these roles as follows:

1. The *encourager* praises, commends, agrees with, and accepts the contributions of others. He invites the participation of other members by indicating warmth, understanding, and acceptance of their ideas, suggestions, and views.

2. The *harmonizer* mediates differences among other members, attempts to reconcile disagreements, and relieves tension in conflict situations through minimizing differences, focusing on compatible points, joking, or pouring oil on the troubled water.

3. The *compromiser* operates from within a conflict in which his idea or position is involved. He may offer compromise by yielding status, admitting his error, or by disciplining himself to meet others halfway.

4. The *gatekeeper and expediter* attempts to keep communication channels open by encouraging or facilitating the participation of others. He may also monitor the length and number of contributions to accommodate participation by all members.

5. The *standard setter* presents standards for the group's functional achievement level or applies standards in evaluating the quality of group processes.

6. The *group observer and commentator* is vigilant of group process and feeds the accumulated data, along with the interpretations, into the group's evaluation of its own procedures.

7. The *follower* goes along with the movement and activity of the group, functioning rather like an audience by more or less passively accepting the ideas and decisions of the others.

INDIVIDUAL ROLES

These roles differ from the group-centered roles in that they are individual-centered roles. Within these seven roles members' concerns and interests are not centered on the good of the group as a whole but on meeting their own individual needs. The behaviors consistent with these roles are often disruptive to group progress because of antagonism to the group building and group maintenance roles. The seven roles are:

1. The *aggressor* may work in many ways. He may deflate the status of others, express disapproval of the values, acts, or feelings of others, attack the group as a whole, joke aggressively, take credit for the contributions of others, or generally try to put members down.

2. The *blocker* tends to be negativistic and stubbornly resistant, disagreeing and opposing without or beyond reason. He may dig his heels in by attempting to maintain or bring back an issue after the group has rejected or bypassed it.

3. The *recognition seeker* uses various means to call attention to himself. Whether through boasting, reporting on personal achievements, acting in unusual ways, or being overtalkative, his principal message is, "Pay attention to me."

4. The *playboy* makes a display of his lack of interest and involvement in the group's processes. This may take the form of cynicism, nonchalance, horseplay, and any other behaviors that convey the message, "I'm just along for the ride."

5. The *dominator* tries to assert authority or superiority in manipulating the group or certain members of the group. This domination may take the form of flattery, of asserting a superior status by having all the answers, giving directions authoritatively, and by not listening to, or interrupting, the contributions of others.

6. The *self-confessor* expresses personal feelings and problems to the exclusion of other types of input. He has difficulty functioning in the here-and-now with the group and tends to focus on the there-and-then.

7. The *arguer* has a strong need to disagree. He continues to present opposing views even when the rest of the members have reached agreement.

The group roles just presented will not be as clearly delineated in a psychotherapy group as they are in a task or social group. This is because decisions are frequently required for the latter groups to proceed and progress, and thus a consensus of opinion may be needed or specific actions may be in order. This variety of activity and interaction allows and calls for more variety in roles than does a straight discussion. Since occupational therapists frequently run task groups or task-discussion groups, becoming familiar with the above roles can be very helpful in observing and analyzing the process in the group. Certain roles, such as the task roles, are likely to emerge more definitively during the task part of a group and decline during the discussion section. During a discussion group or the discussion part of a group, members are apt to function more in individual roles. Also, the leader-therapist may observe that some members participate actively in a task setting but participate minimally during discussions, especially if the discussion revolves around feelings. Observation of these changes in behaviors can form feedback to the members and may be the basis for members' increasing their self-awareness.

Benne and Sheats (1948) note that the combination and balance of member roles is a function of the group's stage of progress and development. In a newly formed group you are likely to observe more task roles, but as the group matures and members become familiar with one another and the purpose of the group, more group-centered roles will emerge. In therapeutic groups where members are grappling with personal problems and expecting help, they may try to meet their needs through functioning in more individual roles. On the other hand, if they are not ready to face their problems, they may avoid bringing attention to themselves by functioning in "follower" or "gatekeeper" roles. In this way, by focusing on the group and other members, they prevent notice themselves and are likely to be acknowledged as agreeable group members. Since it is unwieldy to observe all 26 member roles when analyzing your group, it is useful to combine some and omit others that are very closely related. A suggested format is shown in Figure 12-2.

The names of group members are written across the top of the form in Figure 12-2. Each time they participate in the group a tick is marked in the box under their name beside the member role that most closely describes the context of their contribution. This is not an easy exercise because as you are taking a second or two to evaluate the content of what a member said in order to record it, another member is often responding. Usually though, you can identify and record sufficient observations to obtain a profile of the group that can be useful in your analysis of the group process. You may find it is too distracting to record on the observation form throughout the entire session. In this case it can still be helpful to use it for a portion of the group or for one or two time segments only, for example, the first and last 10-minute segments. This practice of completing a group profile is recommended for new leader-therapists or experienced leader-therapists working with a new group. It helps new leader-therapists focus on the process of the group by examining the various roles that members play. It can also be useful in evaluating the progress or change in the functioning of individual members from session to session. (If possible, completion of a group profile is actually better carried out by an outside observer rather than by the leader-therapist.) As leader-therapists gain experience, they become familiar enough with the roles to be able to identify the member roles without the form. Similar to the way an experienced therapist computes a mental status examination, without having the specific headings laid out in front of her, the leader-therapist becomes skilled in the observation of her group.

SUMMARY

Planning for a therapeutic group necessitates the same attention to detail that is required in the planning of any other type of group. Consideration must be given to and answers determined for who, why, what, when, and where questions. Size is an important factor and since the level of interaction among members is inversely related to number, it is suggested that the preferred membership number be between four and seven.

Based on the fact that we all live and work in a heterogeneous world (which is becoming more and more so) it is believed that heterogeneous groups offer varied experiences and more realistic environments for the members. Even

OBSERVER'S GUIDE					
MEMBERS					
TASK ROLES					
INITIATOR/ CONTRIBUTOR					
INFORMATION/ OPINION SEEKER					
INFORMATION/ OPINION GIVER					
COORDINATOR/ ORIENTOR					
ENERGIZER					
MAINTENANCE ROLES					
ENCOURAGER/ SUPPORTER					
HARMONIZER/ COMPROMISER					
GATEKEEPER/ EXPEDITER					
FOLLOWER					
INDIVIDUAL ROLES					
BLOCKER					
RECOGNITION SEEKER					
DOMINATOR/ AGGRESSOR					
OUT OF FIELD/ ARGUMENTATIVE					

Figure 12-2. Member role observation form.

groups that have been for the most part highly homogeneous in membership, such as a cooking group, are now considered appropriate for a combination of age groups from both sexes.

In a heterogeneous group, members will be found to function in a variety of roles, which can be categorized as task, individual, and group building and maintenance roles. To be familiar with the attitudes and behaviors of members as they carry out these roles and to have an understanding of how the different roles can affect the overall process is an important aspect of being an effective leader-therapist. Focusing on the presence or absence of certain roles can be very enlightening in group analysis. For example, the reason that a group lacks cohesion and is not developing may be attributed in part to the finding that the members all tend to function only in individual roles. It is usually the case that having a mix of member roles results in a more productive and stimulating group. New members will bring new roles, feedback may alter roles, and reinforcement is likely to perpetuate roles.

CHAPTER 13

Group Activities

He started to sing
As he tackled the thing
That couldn't be done,
And he did it.
— EDGAR A. GUEST

Activities have long been the basic tools of treatment for occupational therapists (Allen, 1987; Mosey, 1972; Williamson, 1982) and have been widely used in the treatment of both physical and psychological dysfunction (Levine, 1987). In both spheres the basic premise that *purposeful activity* is a motivating factor to performance has been promoted by occupational therapists. In pointing out that the meaning of purposeful activity has not been clearly delineated in the literature, Steinbeck (1986) goes on to define it as "an activity, task or process in which the individual actively focuses on the achievement of a goal inherent in the activity" (p. 530). He then clarifies that in choosing an activity for a client, the therapist bases her selection on the premise that the client will find the activity sufficiently satisfying to sustain performance. Satisfaction is a key ingredient in motivating clients to perform and then to reap the benefits of their performance, that is, the achievement of a goal or a product (Miller & Nelson, 1987).

The selection of appropriate and satisfying activities for clients is a cornerstone of the practice of occupational therapy. To be proficient in selecting appropriate and satisfying activities the therapist must first define the activity and then become familiar with the activity. The latter can be accomplished by observing or preferably engaging in the activity. Once the therapist is familiar with the activity she is able to complete an analysis of the activity with knowledge and skill (Mosey, 1986). The therapist must go through this process whether the activity is to be used in individual therapy or as a task in small group therapy. In either case the therapist must have a thorough understanding of the innate features, such as the how, when, and where of the activity (Allen, 1987). She must then match these aspects of the activity with the abilities and needs of the client. For example, the *how* of an activity refers to the number of objects or concepts that are required to do an activity. Knowing this the therapist must then decide whether or not the client is able to manipulate or incorporate that many objects or concepts. The *when* and *where* of an activity are obvious but nonetheless important.

Most occupational therapists use activity groups (Duncombe & Howe, 1985) in a wide variety of treatment settings (Steffan & Nelson, 1987). Activity groups provide a setting for learning and accomplishing goals that cannot be achieved in individual therapy (Henry, Nelson, & Duncombe, 1984). As in individual therapy, the tasks or activities employed in a group setting must be selected with care and attention. Several writers have emphasized the therapeutic value of clients engaging in activities of their own choice (Burke, 1977; Howe, 1986; Kuenstler, 1976), but the leader-therapist tends to be the prime selector of tasks in activity groups. Before this point is reached, however, other decisions must first be made regarding each client, namely, determining the initial general treatment program, including treatment modalities.

Sometimes all treatment decisions, even specific group selections, are made by the team. In other facilities referrals are made with or without specific goals. Still other situations operate with blanket referrals. In this last case the occupational therapist will, through formal or informal assessment procedures or both, determine the needs, strengths, and problem areas of the client. Based on these findings she will then formulate an appropriate treatment program which may include assigning the client to various available groups. One of these, for example, might be a cooking group. It is in this environment (the cooking group) that the leader-therapist selects specific activities, although clients can (and it is recommended) be offered choices: snacks versus lunches, lunches versus dinners, items for the menu, types of desserts, and so on.

In selecting a task, the leader-therapist must carry out the same comprehensive task analysis as she would in one-to-one therapy to determine if the activity will be appropriate for the level of functioning of the members of the group. It is very important for a group session to close with the members feeling that they have had a productive and successful experience. They need to leave with a sense of achievement, completion, and competency. Fidler and Fidler (1978) affirm that many clients have had limited "action-learning," and for them, venturing into an activity or task is risky if they fear the undertaking may ultimately demonstrate their incompetence. This is emphasized by Bandura, Jeffrey, and Gajdos (1975) who point out that "powerful success experiences . . . attenuate fearfulness and instill positive attitudes" (p. 151).

In addition to ensuring success, the leader-therapist must determine whether the task will enable the group members to meet their individual goals as well as meet the goals of the group. Another factor that is sometimes ignored but should be considered is the interests of the clients (Kremer, Nelson, & Duncombe, 1984). The leader-therapist should ask and answer the question, "Are the members likely to like the activity?" In conjunction with considering the members' interests, the leader-therapist would be wise to also ask herself, "Does the inherent structure of this activity allow members opportunities to be creative?" Creativity has been emphasized as an important component in the successful use of activities (Cynkin, 1979). The answer to these questions will have some bearing on the decision she makes. The inherent interactive components of a task are also important (Nelson, Peterson, Smith, Boughton, & Whalen, 1988). Some tasks require members to share materials, work in pairs, take turns, work individually, or may even require a single member to be briefly excluded (i.e., he must close his eyes or leave the room). The last, particularly, may be a requisite of certain games but may be counterindicated for some members (i.e., members who are paranoid or who have fragile self-esteem). Summarized, the following six factors should be considered in the selection of a group task or activity:

1. Is the task seen to be purposeful?
2. Do the group members have the abilities to complete the task?
3. Will the task be facilitative in moving the members toward their goals?
4. Will the members like the task?
5. Does the task allow for creative efforts?
6. Are the inherent interactive components appropriate for all the members?

An additional factor that should be addressed in this selection process is whether the principal purpose of the activity is that it serve as a catalyst. Some tasks will have inherent properties in keeping with the group's goals. Other tasks may not have goal-specific properties but are selected for the value of the involvement and process required to complete the task. The manner in which the group is conducted will partially depend on which of these two types of tasks has been selected. If the task has relevant content, such as in cooking or assertiveness training, it is more likely that the leader-therapist will choose to deal with issues as they arise. In this way members are able to learn and correct skills as they participate. If the task is serving mainly as a catalyst, for example, to precipitate a decision making process, the leader-therapist may decide to allow the group to function on its own. While the group is progressing she will observe the process to see how the members approach, participate, make decisions, and interact while completing the task. The process is valuable as it incorporates many functional behaviors that are required in normal day-to-day living. Practicing and learning these behaviors are the primary goals of the experience.

The guided discussion by the leader-therapist during the activity or following completion of the activity will encourage members to examine these issues and facilitate awareness of individual roles and behaviors. The experience also allows members to practice or attempt new behaviors that will promote skills (social and communication) essential for improved functioning in their future lives (De Carlo & Mann, 1985). In the other type of group activity where the activity itself has inherent therapeutic value, such as homemaking or assertiveness training, the members not only practice and hone their interaction and communication skills but they learn the additional specific skills of cooking and assertiveness.

It is usually the case that several group sessions are necessary in order to cover a particular topic thoroughly enough to be of benefit to the members. Certainly more sessions than one are required for clients to achieve meaningful degrees of self-awareness or communication. When using a theme or spreading a topic over several sessions, it is necessary to organize the sessions so that they progress in an orderly fashion. Activities must be graded and selected, in keeping with the group's abilities, similar to the way that activities are graded and selected for individual therapy sessions. Since cooking is an activity commonly used in treatment groups by occupational therapists and is an activity valued by psychiatric patients (Kremer, Nelson, & Duncombe, 1984), it will be used here as an example of organization. The general progression of sessions having an overall theme of cooking and meal preparation could be organized along the following lines:

a. Tasks focusing on nutrition guides, dietary considerations, supplies, recipes, meal planning, and preparations for snacks, light lunches, and full-course meals
b. Formulating shopping lists and outings to various stores to compare prices and purchase supplies
c. Preparation of snacks or light lunches (soups, salads, or sandwiches), eating, and cleaning up
d. Baking and preparation of desserts (cookies, puddings, pies), eating or serving others, and cleaning up

e. Preparation of a one-dish main course (chile, bacon and beans, spaghetti, a casserole) setting the table, eating, and cleaning up

f. Preparation of a full-course meal (meat, potatoes, vegetable), setting the table, eating, and cleaning up

It is important to allow time for discussion during or at the close of each session. This enables members to share their feelings and perceptions, give and receive feedback, and generally consolidate their learning from the experience. It may be necessary at times to lengthen the time allotted for a session in order to accommodate the total activity.

METHODOLOGIC ISSUES

INVOLVEMENT OF THE MEMBERS

Try to involve the group members right from the beginning of the session. If the leader-therapist is active for any extended period of time at the outset of a session, it encourages passivity and dependency in the members. Announcements, if any, should be brief and to the point. Activities should be presented fully but concisely. Complicated and involved instructions should be avoided, if possible, as they tend to confuse and arouse anxiety in the members. Even when you want to get some important concepts or points across, first try to get these points from the members. This gives the members a feeling that they know something about the topic or activity and tends to build confidence, which in turn enhances participation. If you want the points written down so members will remember them or if you plan to refer back to them, have a member write the points down on a flip chart or blackboard. In short, whenever possible, involve a group member!

One technique, referred to in Chapter 1, that is particularly effective in involving members is role playing. As a learning technique role playing evolved from the practice of psychodrama and is now used in a wide variety of fields. Because it is an active technique it tends to involve members more than do the passive verbal techniques. Role plays can be simple, as in learning the social skills of introduction shown in Figure 13-1, or they can be complex, as in role playing in a more composite situation. Other benefits of role playing in a group setting include (a) allowing members to practice new behaviors in a safe environment, (b) providing feedback to the players, (c) gaining insight, (d) increasing sensitivity to the feelings of others, and (e) discovering alternatives (Cabral, 1987).

Each role play generally has four parts: definition of the problem, assuming roles, enactment, and discussion. All four parts are essential for a fertile role play to be completed. Although role playing is appropriate in most groups, some discretion is warranted. Role playing should not be hurried or end without discussion, the latter being where much of the learning takes place. So one

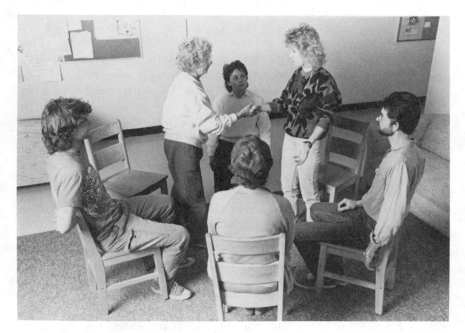

Figure 13-1. Role playing as an action technique.

must be sure that sufficient time is available before embarking on a role-playing activity. Members may not feel comfortable doing role playing if there are high-status persons in the group, although this is not usually a problem in therapeutic groups. Lastly, if there is only one plausible solution to a problem, then role playing to generate alternatives would be meaningless (Cabral, 1987). The spontaneous, visual, imaginative, and here-and-now aspects of role playing all contribute to its dynamic effect.

USE OF VISUAL AIDS

The use of flip charts and blackboards has both advantages and disadvantages. They can be very useful for writing down ideas and points offered by group members so that they can be remembered and seen by all. However, they tend to focus members' attention away from one another and in the process tend to set up a teaching format. As this format becomes accepted members will rely more and more on the leader to "tell them" and less and less on one another. Members may also use the visual aid as a means of avoiding involvement by looking at it rather than interacting with their fellow group members. To help the members focus on the group and one another, it is best to cover the visual aid whenever it is not directly being referred to.

USE OF EXERCISES

Members will interact more if they have something concrete and specific to interact around. Always try to have an exercise or activity relevant to the topic for the members to do. This way they have the results or outcome from the exercise to serve as a catalyst for discussion. Various exercises or activities can be used throughout the group as prompts to further discussion or as a means of introducing a new topic. It is especially important to have some sort of task or activity at the beginning of the group that will serve as a warm-up exercise. Members will come to the group from a variety of situations: a therapy session with a staff member, seeing visitors, having lunch, watching television, taking medication, being alone in their room, or out on recreation. This means they will be in various frames of mind as they enter the session. Starting out with an activity, even a very short one, is a good way to pull them together and help them to refocus on the group and one another. Attempting to facilitate a discussion without an activity is usually left to the psychotherapists. Activity groups tend to be focused and topic-oriented. For example, if the chosen topic is how to handle anger, it is better to have the members make a collage, do a drawing, make a list, or choose symbols that represent how they handle anger than to start by saying, "Today we are going to talk about handling anger," and then wait for the group to begin. The concrete production of lists or pictures gives the members something to talk about and refer to, and will serve as departure points and comparisons for the discussion.

BEING PREPARED

Since every group is unique, one can never be sure of the response that an exercise or activity is going to elicit. Even when the exercise has been used before, the same results or response may not be forthcoming in the next group or in a different session with the same group. An exercise that generated an active discussion in one group may promote only minimal reaction in another group. The leader-therapist should not only be prepared for different responses, but should be prepared with back-up exercises. It can be boring and nonproductive for all involved to try to carry and stretch a discussion that has been exhausted for 10 or 15 minutes more in order to fill up the remaining group time. It is at this point that a new exercise is needed to re-energize the members (and the leader!). It is important that members leave the group with active thoughts and feelings rather than leave feeling lethargic and bored. Members are not likely to feel good about or motivated to return to the group if they leave with negative feelings. Conversely, it can be nonproductive to cut off a lively discussion in order to work in another exercise. The writer has observed therapists initiating an exercise or activity because they had it planned and felt compelled to carry out their plan. Flexibility is the key here. Success lies in not only having back-up exercises but in knowing the right time to fit them into the group.

SUITABLE ACTIVITIES OR TASKS

It was mentioned earlier, but is worth repeating, that the tasks or activities selected for a group must suit the designated topic and the capabilities and interests of the members. An analysis of the activity must be done to determine its suitability to the members in advancing them toward their goals and toward the group's goals.

Literacy is a societal problem that is sometimes overlooked by professionals, but it is an important factor to take into consideration in selecting group tasks or activities. Most paper and pencil exercises require reading and writing in order to complete them and so may be beyond the capabilities of some members. This may come as a surprise to new, bright, highly educated therapists.

Socioeconomic levels must also be considered in the selection of activities. For example, members who come from upper socioeconomic levels are likely to have more money and free time for leisure activities and may see the relevance of leisure or cultural activities more so than members who are out of work or who work long hours for minimal wages. The latter may feel that they have neither the time nor money to engage in the activity in their "real" life, and therefore are not motivated to participate in what they perceive to be an unrealistic endeavor for them.

The masculine-feminine aspects of an activity have some different connotations now than in the past. For example, where a cooking group was usually only considered of interest or value to women, it is now often very appropriate for a mixed group or a men's group. Examples of other topics that should not be compartmentalized as male or female are stress management, time management, assertiveness, life skills, problem solving, and leisure and cultural activities.

LEADERSHIP DEVELOPMENT IN MEMBERS

Therapists enjoying their leadership roles should keep in mind that group members may also enjoy an opportunity to perform as leaders. Whenever members show some leadership skills and aptitudes, try to reinforce their abilities and encourage their efforts. This means, as quoted from Rogers (1951) earlier, that the leader-therapist may relinquish some of her leadership duties to the members. At times this is difficult for the leader-therapist to do, as the emergent member-leader may not be as skilled nor will he carry out the leadership role in what is assessed to be the most effective way. Try to be flexible, tolerant, and accepting in such instances, as the rewards and learning for the members can be substantial. This is not to say that the leader-therapist abandons her leadership role, but rather that she uses it to facilitate leadership and growth in others. Unless there is an obvious deterrent, be open and receptive if members suggest different activities or alternative ways of doing an exercise. Perhaps through problem solving, the member's idea can be adapted to fit the topic and goals of the group.

SUMMARY

Occupational therapists are well aware of the importance of activity analysis in the realm of one-to-one therapy. Analysis of activities is no less important when using task or activity groups. The same meticulous and thorough process of analyzing and evaluating the activity or task to be used in a group is mandatory. Particular attention should be given to the purpose of the activity: Is it to serve mostly as a catalyst or are there important content components to be learned? The determined purpose will direct the leader-therapist and the format for the session. If the main goal of the activity is to generate discussion, you would not have members spend the whole session involved only in the activity. On the other hand, if concrete skills are to be learned, then discussion and feedback are likely to occur as the activity progresses and to continue throughout the entire session. In every group, actively involving the members in the process is a top priority and can be facilitated through warm-up exercises, type of task, participation format, sharing responsibilities, and encouraging emerging leadership.

Challenging as it is, the role of leader-therapist can be an exciting and satisfying endeavor. Enter into it well prepared and with a spirit of enthusiasm, creativity, and diligence, and the outcomes will be rewarding for both you and the members.

BIBLIOGRAPHY

Alcoholics Anonymous World Service (1984). *'Pass it on' the story of Bill Wilson and how the A.A. message reached the world.* New York: Author.

Allen, C. K. (1985). *Occupational therapy for psychiatric diseases: Measurement and management of cognitive disabilities.* Boston: Little, Brown.

Allen, C. K. (1987). Activity: Occupational therapy's treatment method. *American Journal of Occupational Therapy, 41* 563–575.

Allport, F. H. (1920). The influence of the group upon association and thought. *Journal of Experimental Psychology, 3,* 159–182.

Bales, R. F. (1951). *Interaction process analysis.* Cambridge, MA: Addison-Wesley.

Bales, R. F. (1970). *Personality and interpersonal behaviour.* New York: Holt, Rinehart & Winston.

Bales, R. F., Strodtbeck, F. L., Mills, T. M., & Roseborough, M. E. (1951). Channels of communication in small groups. *American Sociological Review, 19,* 461–468.

Bandura, A. (1971). Psychotherapy based upon modeling principles. In A. E. Bergin & S. L. Garfield (Eds.), *Handbook of psychotherapy and behaviour change: An empirical analysis* (pp. 653–708). New York: Wiley.

Bandura, A., Jeffrey, R. W., & Gajdos, E. (1975). Generalizing change through participant modeling with self-directed mastery. *Behavior Research and Therapy, 13,* 141–152.

Banning, M. R., & Nelson, D. L. (1987). The effects of activity-elicited humor and group structure on group cohesion and affective responses. *American Journal of Occupational Therapy, 41,* 510–514.

Barker, L. L. (1981). *Communication* (2nd ed.). Englewood Cliffs, NJ.: Prentice-Hall.

Barker, L. L., Wahlers, K. J., Cegala, D. J., & Kibler, R. J. (1979). *Group in process, an introduction to small groups communication* (1st ed.). Englewood Cliffs, NJ: Prentice-Hall.

Barker, L. L., Wahlers, K. J., Cegala, D. J., & Kibler, R. J., (1983). *Groups in process, an introduction to small groups communication* (2nd ed.). Englewood Cliffs: Prentice-Hall.

Barris, R. (1982). Environmental interactions: An extension of the model of occupation. *American Journal of Occupational Therapy, 36,* 637–644.

Barris, R., & Kielhofner, G. (1986). Beliefs, perspectives, and activities of psychosocial occupational therapy. *American Journal of Occupational Therapy, 40,* 535–541.

Bass, B. M. (1981). *Stodgill's handbook of leadership.* New York: Macmillan.

Battegay, R. (1986). People in groups: Dynamic and therapeutic aspects. *Group, 10,* 131–148.

Beck, A. P. (1981). A study of group phase development and emergent leadership. *Group, 5,* 48–54.

Beck, A. T. (1967). *Depression: Clinical, experimental and theoretical aspects.* New York: Harper & Row.

Beck, A. T. (1976). *Cognitive therapy and emotional disorders.* New York: International Universities Press.

Benjamin, A. (1978). *Behaviour in small groups.* Boston: Houghton Mifflin.

Benne, K. D., & Sheats, P. (1948). Functional roles of group members. *Journal of Social Issues, 4,* 41–49.

Bennis, W. G., & Shepard, H. A. (1978). A theory of group development. In L. P. Bradford (Ed.), *Group development* (2nd ed.), (pp. 13–35). La Jolla, CA: University Associates.

Bernard, H. W. (1974). *Personality: Applying theory.* Boston: Holbrook.

Berne, E. (1966). *Principles of group treatment.* New York: Oxford Press.

Bertalanffy, L. (1968). General system theory — A critical review. In W. Buckley (Ed.), *Modern systems research for the behavioral scientist* (pp. 10–30). Chicago: Aldine.

Bertcher, H. J., and Maple, F. F. (1977). *Creating groups.* Beverly Hills, CA: SAGE.

Bion, W. R. (1961). *Experience in groups.* New York: Basic Books.

Bloch, S., Browning, S., & McGrath, G. (1983). Humour in group psychotherapy. *British Journal of Medical Psychology, 56,* 89–97.

Block, S., & Crouch, E. (1985). *Therapeutic factors in group psychotherapy.* Oxford, England: Oxford University Press.

Block, S., Crouch, E., & Reibstein, J. (1981). Therapeutic factors in group psychotherapy. *Archives of General Psychiatry, 38,* 519–526.

Blumberg, A., & Golembiewski, R. T. (1976). *Learning and change in groups.* Baltimore: Penguin Books.

Bonner, H. (1959). *Group dynamics: Principles and applications.* New York: Ronald Press.

Bonney, W. C., Randall, D. A., Jr., & Cleveland, J. D. (1986). An analysis of client-perceived curative factors in a therapy group of former incest victims. *Small Group Behavior, 17,* 303–321.

Braaten, L. J. (1974/1975). Developmental phases of encounter groups and related intensive groups: A critical review of models and a new proposal. *Interpersonal Development, 5,* 112-129.

Bradford, L. P. (1964a). Trainer-intervention: Case episodes. In L. P. Bradford, J. R. Gibb, & K. D. Benne (Eds.), *T-group theory and laboratory method.* (pp. 136–167). New York: Wiley.

Bradford L. P. (1964b). Membership and the learning process. In L. P. Bradford, J. R. Gibb, & K. D. Benne (Eds.), *T-group theory and laboratory method.* (pp. 190–215). New York: Wiley.

Bradford, L. P. (1978a). Group formation and development. In L. P. Bradford (Ed.), *Group development* (2nd ed.), (pp. 4–12). La Jolla, CA: University Associates.

Bradford, L. P. (1978b). The case of the hidden agenda. In L. P. Bradford (Ed.), *Group development* (2nd ed.), (pp. 84–94). La Jolla, CA: University Associates.

Bradlee, L. (1984). The use of groups in short-term psychiatric settings. *Occupational Therapy in Mental Health, 4,* 47–57.

Brilhart, J. K. (1974). *Effective group discussion.* Dubuque, IA: Wm. C. Brown.

Buchanan, D. C. (1978). Group therapy for chronic physically ill patients. *Psychosomatics, 19,* 425–431.

Burgoon, M., Heston, J. K., & McCroskey, J. (1974). *Small group communication: A functional approach.* New York: Holt, Rinehart & Winston.

Burke, J. P. (1977). A clinical perspective on motivation: Pawn vs. origin. *American Journal of Occupational Therapy, 31,* 254–258.

Cabral, R. J. (1987). Role playing as a group intervention. *Small Group Behavior, 18,* 470–482.

Castore, G. (1962). Number of verbal interrelationships as a determinant of group size. *Journal of Abnormal and Social Psychology, 64,* 456–457.

Checkland, P. (1981). *Systems thinking, systems practice.* New York: Wiley.

Comrey, A. L., & Staats, C. K. (1955). Group performance in a cognitive task. *Journal of Applied Psychology, 39,* 354–356.

Cooper, J. B., & McGaugh, J. L. (1969). Leadership. In C. A. Gibb (Ed.), *Leadership* (pp. 242–253). Harmondsworth, England: Penguin Books.

Corey, G. (1982). *Theory and practice of counselling and psychotherapy* (2nd ed.). Monterey, CA: Brooks/Cole.

Corey, G., & Corey, S. (1982). *Groups: Process and practice* (2nd ed.). Monterey, CA: Brooks/Cole.

Corey G., Corey, M., & Callanan, P. (1979). *Professional and ethical issues in counselling and psychotherapy.* Monterey, CA: Brooks/Cole.

Cunningham, L. L., & Carol, L. N. (1986). Leaders and leadership: 1985 and beyond. *Proceedings of symposium, occupational therapy education: Target 2000.* Rockville, MD: American Occupational Therapy Association.

Cynkin, S. (1979). *Occupational therapy: Toward health through activities.* Boston: Little, Brown.

De Carlo, J. J., & Mann, W. C. (1985). The effectiveness of verbal versus activity groups in improving self-perceptions of interpersonal communication skills. *American Journal of Occupational Therapy, 39,* 20–27.

Derlega, V. J., & Chaikin, A. L. (1975). *Sharing intimacy: what we reveal to others and why.* Englewood Cliffs, NJ: Prentice-Hall.

Diedrich, R., & Dye, A. (Eds.). (1972). *Group procedures: Purposes, processes and outcomes, selected readings for the counselor.* Boston: Houghton Mifflin.

Dimock, H. G. (1985a). *How to observe your group* (2nd ed.). Guelph, Ont., Canada: University of Guelph.

Dimock, H. G. (1985b). *How to analyze and evaluate group growth* (2nd ed.). Guelph, Ont., Canada: University of Guelph.

Dimock, H. G. (1985c). *Planning group development* (2nd ed.). Guelph, Ont., Canada: University of Guelph.

Donohue, M. (1982). Designing activities to develop a women's identification group. *Occupational Therapy in Mental Health, 2,* 1–19.

Duncombe, L. W., & Howe, M. C. (1985). Group work in occupational therapy: A survey of practice. *American Journal of Occupational Therapy, 39,* 163–170.

Dunphy, D. C. (1972). *The primary group: A handbook for analysis and field research:* New York: Meredith.

Egan, G. (1976). *Interpersonal living.* Monterey, CA: Brooks/Cole.

Egan, G. (1983). Some suggested rules for confrontation. In H. H. Blumberg, A. P. Hare, V. Kent, & M. F. Davies (Eds.), *Small groups and social interaction* (pp. 237–238). New York: Wiley.

Ellis, A. (1974). The group as agent in facilitating change toward rational thinking and appropriate emoting. In A. Jacobs & W. W. Spradlin (Eds.), *The group as agent of change* (pp. 100–115). New York: Behavioral Publications.

Erickson. R. C. (1986). Heterogeneous groups: A legitimate alternative. *Group, 10,* 21–26.

Erikson, E. H. (1963). *Childhood and society* (2nd ed.). New York: Norton.

Fidler, G. S., & Fidler, J. W. (1978). Doing and becoming: Purposeful action and self-actualization. *American Journal of Occupational Therapy, 32,* 305–310.

Fisher, B. A. (1974). *Small group decision making: Communication and the group process.* New York: McGraw-Hill.

Flapan, D., & Fenchel, G. H. (1987). Terminations. *Group, 11,* 131–143.

Freud, S. (1922). *Group psychology and the analysis of the ego.* London: Hogarth Press.

Fried, E. (1972). Basic concepts in group psychotherapy. In H. I. Kaplan & B. J. Sadock (Eds.), *The evolution of group therapy* (pp. 27–50). New York: E.P. Dutton.

Funk and Wagnalls standard college dictionary (1982). Toronto: Fitzhenry & Whiteside.

Furst, W. (1975). Homogeneous versus heterogeneous groups. In M. Rosenbaum & M. M. Berger (Eds.), *Group psychotherapy and group function* (pp. 409–412). New York: Basic Books.

Gallogly, V., & Levine, B. (1979). Co-therapy. In B. Levine (Ed.), *Group psychotherapy: Practice and development* (pp. 296–305). Englewood Cliffs, NJ: Prentice-Hall.

Geller, L. (1982). The failure of self-actualization theory: A critique of Carl Rogers and Abraham Maslow. *Journal of Humanistic Psychology, 22,* 56–73.

Gemmill, G. (1986). The mythology of the leader role in small groups. *Small Group Behavior, 17,* 41–50.

Getty, C., & Shannon, A. M. (1969). Co-therapy as an egalitarian relationship. *American Journal of Nursing, 69,* 767–771.

Gibb, C. A. (Ed.), (1969a). *Leadership.* Harmondsworth, England: Penguin Books.

Gibb, C. A. (1969b). Leadership. In G. Linsey & E. Aronson (Eds.), *The handbook of social psychology* (2nd ed.), (pp. 205–282). Reading, MA: Addison-Wesley.

Gibb, J. R. (1969). Dynamics of leadership. In W. B. Eddy, W. W. Burke, V. A. Dupre, & O. P. South (Eds.), *Behavioral science and the manager's role* (pp. 121–135). Washington, DC: NTL Institute for Applied Behavioral Science.

Gibb, J. R., & Gibb L. M. (1978). The group as a growing organism. In L. P. Bradford (Ed.), *Group development* (pp. 104–116). La Jolla, CA: University Associates.

Ginsberg, C. (1984). Toward a more somatic understanding of self. *Journal of Humanistic Psychology, 24,* 66–92.

Glasser, W. (1965). *Reality therapy.* New York: Harper & Row.

Glasser, W., & Zunin, L. M. (1979). Reality therapy. In R. J. Corsini (Ed.), *Current psychotherapies* (pp. 302–339). Itasca, IL: F. E. Peacock.

Goldman, M. (1965). A comparison of individual and group performance for varying combinations of initial ability. *Journal of Personality and Social Psychology, 1,* 210–216.

Goldstein, A. P., & Myers, C. R. (1986). Relationship enhancement methods. In F. H. Kanfer & A. P. Goldstein (Eds.), *Helping people change: A textbook of methods* (3rd. ed.), (pp. 19–65). New York: Pergamon Press

Grieger, R., & Boyd. J. (1980). *Rational-emotive therapy: A skills-based approach.* New York: Van Nostrand Reinhold.

Haaga, D. A., & Davison, G. C. (1986). Cognitive change methods. In F. H. Kanfer & A. P. Goldstein (Eds.), *Helping people change: A textbook of methods* (3rd ed.), (pp. 236–282). Elmsford, NY: Pergamon Press.

Haley, J. (1976). *Problem-solving therapy.* San Francisco: Jossey-Bass.

Hall, A. D., & Fagen, R. E. (1968). Definition of a system. In W. Buckley (Ed.), *Modern systems research for the behavioral scientist* (pp. 81–92). Chicago: Aldine.

Hall, E. T. (1966). *The hidden dimension.* Garden City, NY: Doubleday.

Halperin, D. (1987). The self-help group: The mental health professional's role. *Group, 11,* 47–53.

Handelsman, M. M., & Snyder, C. R. (1982). Is "rejected" feedback really rejected?: Effects of informativeness on reactions to positive and negative personality feedback. *Journal of Personality, 50,* 168–179.

Hansen, J. C., Warner, R. W., & Smith, E.M. (1976). *Group counseling: Theory and process.* Chicago: Rand McNally.

Hare, A. P. (1976). *Handbook of small group research* (2nd ed.). New York: Free Press.

Heap, K. (1977). *Group theory for social workers.* Oxford: Pergamon Press.

Henry, A. D., Nelson, D. L., & Duncombe, L. W. (1984). Choice making in group and individual activity. *American Journal of Occupational Therapy, 38,* 245–251.

Herbert, E. L., & Trist, E. L. (1953). The institution of an absent leader by a students' discussion group. *Human Relations, 6,* 215–248.

Howe, M. C. (1986). An occupational therapy activity group. *American Journal of Occupational Therapy, 22,* 176–179.

Howe, M. C., & Schwartzberg, S. L. (1986). *A functional approach to group work in occupational therapy.* Philadelphia: J. B. Lippincott.

Janov, A. (1972). *The primal revolution.* New York: Simon & Schuster.

Jennings, E. E. (1960). *An anatomy of leadership: Princes, heroes, and superman.* New York: Harper.

Johnson, D. W., & Johnson, F. P. (1982). *Joining together: group therapy and group skills* (2nd ed.). Englewood Cliffs, NJ: Prentice-Hall.

Johnston, M. T. (1987). Occupational therapists and the teaching of cognitive behavioral skills. *Occupational Therapy in Mental Health, 7,* 69–81.

Jordon, N. (1968). *Themes in speculative psychology.* London: Tavistock.

Kanfer, F. H., & Goldstein, A. P. (1986). *Helping people change: A textbook of methods.* Elmsford, NY: Pergamon Press.

Kaplan, H. I., & Sadock, B. J. (1985). *Modern synopsis of comprehensive textbook of psychiatry/IV* (4th ed.). Baltimore, MD: Williams & Wilkins.

Kaplan, K. L. (1986). The directive group: Treatment for psychiatric patients with a minimum level of functioning. *American Journal of Occupational Therapy, 40,* 474–481.

Kell, C. L., & Corts, P. R. (1980). *Fundamentals of effective group communication.* New York: Macmillan.

Kielhofner, G. (1985). *A model of human occupation: Theory and application.* Baltimore, MD.: Williams & Wilkins.

Knowles, M., & Knowles, H. (1972). *Introduction to group dynamics* (rev. ed.). New York: Association Press.

Kottler, J. A. (1983). *Pragmatic group leadership.* Monterey, CA: Brooks/Cole.

Kremer, E. R. H., Nelson, D. L., & Duncombe, L. W. (1984). Effects of selected activities on affective meaning in psychiatric patients. *American Journal of Occupational Therapy, 38,* 522–528.

Kreps, G. L., & Thornton, B. C. (1984). *Health communication.* New York: Longman.

Kuenstler, G. (1976). A planning group for psychiatric outpatients. *American Journal of Occupational Therapy, 30,* 634–639.

Lakin, M. (1983). Experiential helping groups. In H. H. Blumberg, A. P. Hare, V. Kent, & M. Davies (Eds.), *Groups and social interaction* (pp. 209–226). New York: Wiley.

Latham, Van M. (1987). Task type and group motivation. *Small Group Behavior, 18,* 56–71.

Levine, B. (1979). *Group psychotherapy: practice and development.* Englewood Cliffs, NJ: Prentice-Hall.

Levine, R. E. (1987). The influence of the arts-and-crafts movement on the professional status of occupational therapy. *American Journal of Occupational Therapy, 41,* 248–254.

Lewin, K. (1947). Group decisions and social change. In T. M. Newcomb & E. L. Hartley (Eds.), *Readings in social psychology* (pp. 64–82). New York: Holt, Rinehart & Winston.

Lewin, K., Lippitt, R., & White, R. K. (1939). Patterns of aggressive behavior in experimentally created "social climates." *Journal of Social Psychology, 10,* 271–299.

Lewis, P. (1987). Therapeutic change in groups: An interactional perspective. *Small Group Behavior, 18,* 548–556.

Lieberman, M. A. (1983). Comparative analyses of change mechanisms in groups. In H. H. Blumberg, A. P. Hare, & M. Davies (Eds.), *Small groups and social interaction* (pp. 239–252). New York: Wiley.

Lieberman, M. A., Yalom, I. D., & Miles, M. B. (1973). *Encounter groups: First facts.* New York: Basic Books.

Lifton, W. R. (1972). *Groups: facilitating individual growth and societal change.* New York: Wiley.

Long, L., & Cope, C. (1980). Curative factors in a male felony offender group. *Small Group Behavior, 11,* 389–398.

Loomis, M. E. (1979). *Group process for nurses.* St. Louis: Mosby.

Low, M., & Low, P. (1975). Treatment of married couples in a group run by a husband and wife. *International Journal of Group Psychotherapy, 25,* 54–56.

Luft, J. (1984). *Group processes, an introduction to group dynamics* (3rd ed.). Palo Alto, CA: Mayfield.

MacDevitt, J. W., & Sanislow, C. (1987). Curative factors in offenders. *Group, 18,* 72–81.

MacKenzie, K. R. (1987). Therapeutic factors in group psychotherapy: A contemporary view. *Group, 11,* 26–34.

MacLennan. B. W. (1965). Co-therapy. *International Journal of Group Psychotherapy, 15,* 154–166.

Mahler, C. (1969). *Group counseling in the schools.* New York: Houghton Mifflin.

Mann, R. D. (1967). *Interpersonal styles and group development.* New York: Wiley.

Markowitz, M., & Kadis, A. L. (1972). Short-term analytic treatment of married couples in a group by a therapist couple. In C. J. Sager & H. S. Kaplan (Eds.), *Progress in group and family therapy.* New York: Brunner/Mazel.

Maslow, A. H. (1962). *Toward a psychology of being.* Princeton, NJ.: Van Nostrand Reinhold.

Matthews, K. A., Batson, C. D., Horn, J., & Rosenman, R. H. (1981). "Principles in his nature which interest him in the fortune of others . . . ": The heritability of empathic concern for others. *Journal of Personality, 49,* 237–247.

McAdams, D. P., Jackson, J., & Kirshnit, C. (1984). Looking, laughing, and smiling in dyads as a function of intimacy, motivation and reciprocity. *Journal of Personality, 52,* 261–273.

McFall, R. M., & Marston, A. R. (1970). An experimental investigation of behavior rehearsal in assertive training. *Journal of Abnormal Psychology, 76,* 295–303.

Meador, B. D., & Rogers, C. R. (1979). Person-centered therapy. In R. J. Corsini (Ed.), *Current psychotherapies* (pp. 131–184). Itasca, IL: F. E. Peacock.

Mehrabian, A. (1971). *Silent messages.* Belmont, CA: Wadsworth.

Miller, L., & Nelson, D. L. (1987). Dual-purpose activity versus single-purpose activity in terms of duration on task, exertion level, and affect. *Occupational Therapy in Mental Health, 7,* 55–67.

Monane, J. H. (1967). *Sociology of human systems.* New York: Appleton-Century-Crofts.

Moreno, J. L. (1957). *The first book on group psychotherapy.* New York: Beacon House.

Mosey, A. C. (1970). The concept and use of developmental groups. *American Journal of Occupational Therapy, 24,* 272–275.

Mosey, A. C. (1972). *Activity therapy.* New York: Raven Press.

Mosey, A. C. (1986). *Psychosocial components of occupational therapy.* New York: Raven Press.

Mullen, H., & Sanguiliano, I. (1960). Multiple psychotherapeutic practice: Preliminary report. *American Journal of Psychotherapy, 14,* 550–565.

Napier, R. W., & Gershenfeld, M. K. (1973). *Groups: Theory and experience.* Boston: Houghton Mifflin.

Nelson, A., Mackenthun, D., Bloesch, A., Milan, A., Unrein, M., & Hill, K. (1956). A preliminary report on a study in group occupational therapy. *American Journal of Occupational Therapy, 10,* 254–258, 262–263, 271.

Nelson, D. L., Peterson, C., Smith, D. A., Boughton, J. A., & Whalen, G. M. (1988). Effects of project versus parallel groups on social interaction and affective responses in senior citizens. *American Journal of Occupational Therapy, 42,* 23–29.

New Lexicon Webster's Dictionary (1987). New York: Lexicon Publications.

Nixon, H. L. (1979). *The small group.* Englewood Cliffs, NJ: Prentice-Hall.

Orme, M. E. J. (1987). Uses of humour in instruction. *Reflections, 25,* 1–4.

Palazzolo, C. S. (1981). *Small groups: An introduction.* New York: Van Nostrand Reinhold.

Pellegrini, R. J. (1971). Some effects of seating position on social perception. *Psychological Reports, 28,* 887–893.

Pedretti, L. W. (1985). *Occupational therapy practice skills for physical dysfunction* (2nd ed.). St. Louis: Mosby.

Penland, P. R., & Fine, S. F. (1974). *Group dynamics and individual development.* New York: Marcel Dekker.

Pfeiffer, J. W., & Jones, J. E. (1972). *Annual handbook for group facilitators.* La Jolla, CA: University Associates.

Pollak, G. K. (1975). *Leadership of discussion groups.* New York: Spectrum.

Posthuma, B. W. (1972). Personal development and occupational therapy. *American Journal of Occupational Therapy, 26,* 88–90.

Posthuma, B. W. (1976). A deprivation experience. *Canadian Journal of Occupational Therapy, 43,* 129–130.

Posthuma, B. W. (1985). Learning to touch. *Canadian Journal of Occupational Therapy, 52,* 189–193.

Posthuma, B. W., & Posthuma, A. B. (1972). The effect of a small-group experience on occupational therapy students. *American Journal of Occupational Therapy, 26,* 415–418.

Posthuma, A. B., & Posthuma, B. W. (1973). Some observations on encounter group casualties. *Journal of Applied Behavioural Science, 9,* 595–608.

Potter, D., & Anderson, M. P. (1970). *Discussion: A guide to effective practice.* Belmont, CA: Wadsworth.

Prazoff, M., Joyce, A. S., & Azim, H. F. A. (1986). Brief crises group psychotherapy: One therapist's model. *Group, 10,* 34–40.

Purtilo, R. (1978). *Health professional/patient interaction.* Philadelphia: W. B. Saunders.

Rabin, H. (1967). How does co-therapy compare with regular group therapy? *American Journal of Psychotherapy, 21,* 244–255.

Rapoport, A. (1968). Forward. In W. Buckley (Ed.), *Modern systems research for the behavioral scientist* (pp. xiii–xxii). Chicago: Aldine

Remocker, A. J., & Storch, E. T. (1979). *Action speaks louder, A handbook of nonverbal group techniques* (2nd ed.). Edinburgh: Churchill Livingstone.

Rice, D. G., Razin, A. M., & Gurman, A. S. (1976). Spouses as co-therapists: "Style" variables and implications for patient-therapist matching. *Journal of Marriage and Family Counselling, 2,* 55–62.

Rogers, C. R. (1951). *Client-centered therapy.* Boston: Houghton Mifflin.

Rogers, C. R. (1961). *On becoming a person.* Boston: Houghton Mifflin.

Rogers, C. R. (1985). Comment on Slack's article. *Journal of Humanistic Psychology, 25,* 43–44.

Rose, S. D. (1986). Group methods. In F. H. Kanfer & A. P. Goldstein (Eds.), *Helping people change: A textbook of methods* (3rd. ed.), (pp. 437–469). Elmsford, NY: Pergamon.

Rosenbaum, L. L., & Rosenbaum, W. B. (1971). Morale and productivity consequences of group leadership style, stress, and type of task. *Journal of Applied Psychology, 55,* 343–348.

Rosenbaum, M. (1973). Co-therapy. In M. Rosenbaum & M. Berger (Eds.), *Group psychotherapy and group function.* (rev. ed.), (pp. 389–408). New York: Basic Books.

Rosenbaum, M. (1976). Group psychotherapy. In M. Rosenbaum & A. Snadowsky (Eds.), *The intensive group experience* (pp. 1–49). New York: Free Press.

Rosenbaum, M., & Berger, M. M. (1975). *Group psychotherapy and group function* (rev ed.). New York: Basic Books.

Rudestam, K. E. (1982). *Experiential groups in theory and practice.* Monterey, CA: Brooks/Cole.

Ruitenbeek, H. M. (1970). *The new group therapies.* New York: Avon Books.

Russell, A., & Russell, L. (1979). The uses and abuses of co-therapy. *Journal of Marital and Family Therapy, 5,* 39–46.

Sadock, B. J., & Kaplan, H. I. (1972). Selection of patients and the dynamic and structural organization of the group. In H. I. Kaplan & B. J. Sadock (Eds.), *The evolution of group therapy* (pp. 119–131). New York: E. P. Dutton.

Samovar, L. A., & Mills, J. (1976). *Oral communication* (3rd. ed.). Dubuque, IA: Wm. C. Brown.

Sampson, E. E., & Marthas, M. (1981). *Group process for the health professions* (2nd ed.). New York: Wiley.

Schroder, H. M., & Harvey, O. J. (1963). Conceptual organization and group structure. In O. J. Harvey (Ed.), *Motivation and social interaction* (pp. 134–166). New York: Ronald Press.

Schultz, B. (1986). Communication correlates of perceived leaders in the small group. *Small Group Behavior, 17,* 51–65.

Schwartzberg, S. L., Howe, M. C., & McDermott, A. (1982). A comparison of three treatment group formats for facilitating social interaction. *Occupational Therapy in Mental Health, 2,* 1–17.

Seashore, C. (1974). Time and transition in the intensive group experience. In A. Jacobs & W. W. Spradlin (Eds.), *The group as agent of change.* New York: Behavioral Publications.

Shannon, P. D., & Snortum, J. R. (1965). An activity group's role. *American Journal of Occupational Therapy, 19,* 344–347.

Shapiro, J. L. (1978). *Methods of group psychotherapy: A tradition of innovation.* Itasea, IL: F. E. Peacock.

Shaw, M. E. (1976). *Group dynamics: The psychology of small group behavior* (2nd ed.). New York: McGraw-Hill.

Sherman, S. J., & Fazio, R. H. (1983). Parallels between attitudes and traits as predictors of behavior. *Journal of Personality, 51,* 308–345.

Shoemaker, G. (1987). A study of human relations training groups: Leadership style and outcome. *Small Group Behavior, 18,* 356–366.

Slavson, S. R. (1963). Personality qualifications of a group psychotherapist. *International Journal of Group Psychotherapy, 13,* 411–419.

Smith, P. B. (1980a). *Group processes and personal change.* London: Harper & Row.

Smith, P. B. (Ed.). (1980b). *Small groups and personal change.* London: Methuen.

Smith, P. B., Wood, H., & Smale, G. G. (1980). The usefulness of groups in clinical settings. In P. B. Smith (Ed.), *Small groups and personal change.* New York: Methuen.

Snyder, C. R., Ingram, R. E., Handelsman, M. M., & Wells, D. S. (1982). Desire for personal feedback: Who wants it and what does it mean for psychotherapy? *Journal of Personality, 50,* 316–330.

Sommer, R. (1962). The distance for comfortable conversation: A further study. *Sociometry, 25,* 111–116.

Spotts, J. V. (1969). The problem of leadership: A look at some recent findings of behavioral science research. In W. B. Eddy, W. W. Burke, V. A. Dupre, & O. P. South (Eds.), *Behavioral science and the manager's role* (pp. 136–154). Washington, DC: NTL Institute for Applied Behavioral Science.

Stake, J. E. (1983). Situation and person-centered approaches to promoting leadership behavior in low performance self-esteem women. *Journal of Personality, 51,* 61–77.

Steffan, L. A., & Nelson, D. L. (1987). The effects of tool scarcity on group climate and affective meaning within the context of a stenciling activity. *American Journal of Occupational Therapy, 41,* 449–453.

Steinbeck, T. M. (1986). Purposeful activity and performance. *American Journal of Occupational Therapy, 40,* 529–534.

Steiner, I. D. (1972). *Group process and productivity.* New York: Academic Press.

Stogdill, R. M. (1969). Personal factors associated with leadership: A survey of the literature. In C. A. Gibb (Ed.), *Leadership* (pp. 91–133). Harmondsworth, England: Penguin Books.

Tannenbaum, R., & Schmidt, W. H. (1958). How to choose a leadership pattern. *Harvard Business Review, 36,* 95–101.

Taylor, E. (1988). Anger intervention. *American Journal of Occupational Therapy, 42,* 147–155.

Thompson, S., & Kahn, J. H. (1970). *The group process as a helping technique.* Oxford, England: Pergamon Press.

Tooper, V. O. (1984). Humor as an adjunct to occupational therapy interactions. *Occupational Therapy in Health Care, 1,* 49–59.

Toothman, J. M. (1978). *Conducting the small group experience.* Washington, DC: University Press of America.

Trotzer, J. P. (1977). *The counselor and the group: Integrating theory, training, and practice.* Monterey, CA: Brooks/Cole.

Truax, C. B., & Carkhuff, R. R. (1967). *Toward effective counseling and psychotherapy.* Chicago: Aldine.

Tuckman, B. W. (1965). Developmental sequence in small groups. *Psychological Bulletin, 63,* 384–399.

Tuckman, B. W., & Jensen, M. A. C. (1977). Stages of small group development revisited. *Group and Organization Studies, 2,* 419–427.

Verba, S. (1961). *Small groups and political behaviour: A study of leadership.* Princeton, NJ: Princeton University Press.

Waldinger, R. J. (1986). *Fundamentals of psychiatry.* Washington, DC: American Psychiatric Press.

Watzlawick, P., Beavin, J. H., & Jackson, D. D. (1967). *Pragmatics of human communication.* New York: W. W. Norton.

Whitaker, D. S., & Lieberman, M. A. (1964). *Psychotherapy through the group process.* New York: Authuton Press.

Williams, R. A. (1976). A contract for co-therapist in group psychotherapy. *Journal of Psychosocial Nursing and Mental Health Services, 14,* 11–14.

Williamson, G. G. (1982). A heritage of activity: Development of a theory. *American Journal of Occupational Therapy, 36,* 716–730.

Wolf, A. (1975). Psychoanalysis in groups. In M. Rosenbaum & M. M. Berger (Eds.), *Group psychotherapy and group function* (rev. ed.), (pp. 321–335). New York: Basic Books.

Wolfe, M., & Proshansky, H. (1974). The physical setting as a factor in group function and process. In A. Jacobs & W. Spradlin (Eds.), *The group as agent of change* (pp. 206–227). New York: Behavioral Publications.

Yalom, I. D. (1970). *The theory and practice of groups.* New York: Basic Books.

Yalom, I. D. (1983). *Inpatient group psychotherapy.* New York: Basic Books.

Youcha, I. Z. (1976). Short-term in-patient groups: Formation and beginnings. *Group Process, 7,* 119–137.

Zander, A., Natsoulas, T., & Thomas, E. J. (1978). Personal goals and the group's goals for the member. In L. P. Bradford (Ed.), *Group development* (2nd ed.), (pp. 167–181). La Jolla, CA: University Associates.

Zimet, C. N., & Schneider, C. (1969). Effects of group size on interaction in small groups. *Journal of Social Psychology, 77,* 177–187.

APPENDICES

Appendices A and B contain examples of how to plan and organize a series of group sessions around the central themes of assertiveness and awareness, respectively. Suggested activities and exercises for six sessions on each theme are included. Depending on the functional level of the members the content presented may be appropriate as laid out for six sessions or it may need to be reorganized into additional or fewer sessions.

Recommendations are included as to the types of problems that can be addressed in the sessions. There are some minimal functional requirements that clients must meet in order to benefit from the sessions as they are laid out, and these limitations are included as recommendations for client selection.

The format used here has the general objectives for the overall experience (six sessions) presented at the beginning. In a similar way the leader-therapist will want to formulate specific objectives for each session relative to her group members.

Appendix A

Small Group Program

Theme: Assertiveness

Sessions: Six

Recommendations:

For these problem areas:

1. Anxiety
2. Difficulty speaking spontaneously
3. Low self-esteem
4. Low self-confidence
5. Nonassertive approach to others
6. Aggressive approach to others

For clients who are:

1. Functionally literate
2. Able to interact verbally at least at a minimal level
3. Cognitively alert

Objectives:

1. To improve awareness, recognition, and expression of feelings in an appropriate manner, both verbally and nonverbally
2. To enable differentiation between assertive, nonassertive, and aggressive behavior.
3. To practice assertive rights and responsibilities in order to increase self-respect and self-esteem as well as to gain respect from others
4. To learn basic conversational skills in order to reduce social anxieties
5. To learn appropriate ways of making and refusing requests
6. To learn a problem solving approach to clearer communication through familiarization of the DESC system (i.e., format for an assertive response)
7. To learn coping skills in dealing with manipulation and unfair criticism

Effective Aids:

1. Structured exercises
2. Suggested situations for role plays
3. Printed handouts or manuals
4. Posters
5. Flip chart or blackboard
6. Homework assignments

Topics:

Session 1: Nonassertive behaviors; aggressive behaviors
Session 2: Assertive behaviors; nonverbal components of behaviors
Session 3: Barriers to being assertive; the ABC of emotions
Session 4: Assertiveness rights and responsibilities; principles of assertiveness; the DESC script
Session 5: Broken record; workable compromise
Session 6: Building self-respect; coping with criticism

SESSION 1

NONASSERTIVE BEHAVIOR

The aim of nonassertive behavior is to please others and to *avoid conflict* at any cost. It results in the loss of self-respect. When you are nonassertive what message are you actually conveying to others? (Try to get group members to offer ideas similar to those given below.)
    Nonassertive behavior says, in effect:

"You're O.K, I'm not O.K."
"I don't count."
"My feelings don't matter."
"I don't respect myself."

Exercise 1. This exercise will help you to recognize how often you behave in the following nonassertive ways:

	Always	Often	Sometimes	Never
1. Letting others take the initiative in starting conversations	_____	_____	_____	_____
2. Being unable to refuse requests for your time, energy, or money	_____	_____	_____	_____

3. Failing to express your
   feelings or opinions when
   you would like to do so

4. Not accepting a
   compliment when you
   would like to do so

5. Being unable to give a
   compliment when you
   would like to

6. Letting criticism
   overwhelm you without
   saying anything

7. Having difficulty giving
   criticism or giving a
   compliment

8. Frequently apologizing
   for or justifying your
   behavior to others

Discussion by members of their answers to the examples follows. Figure A-1 exemplifies that nonassertive behavior invites others to "walk over us."

Figure A-1. Nonassertive behavior invites being walked over.

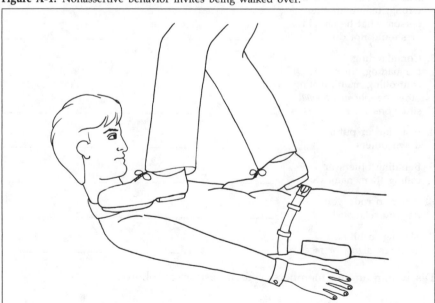

AGGRESSIVE BEHAVIOR

The aim of aggressive behavior is to achieve or maintain control over people or situations. It can cause others to feel humiliated, put down, and angry. When you are being aggressive, what message are you really sending to others? (Try to get members to offer ideas similar to those below.)

Aggressive behavior says in effect:

"I'm O.K., you're not O.K."
"This is what I want, think, or feel. You have no right to want, think, or feel otherwise."
"You don't count."
"I don't respect you."

Exercise 2. Below is a list of some of the ways people behave aggressively. Read the list and in the columns at the right, indicate how frequently you behave aggressively in these ways.

	Always	*Often*	*Sometimes*	*Never*
1. Speaking for others	_____	_____	_____	_____
2. Making judgments on who or what is right or wrong; telling another person what he should or should not do	_____	_____	_____	_____
3. Commanding, persuading, directing, controlling, manipulating other people in *personal* situations	_____	_____	_____	_____
4. Insulting or putting down others	_____	_____	_____	_____
5. Belittling others or calling them names	_____	_____	_____	_____
6. Being so rude you destroy relationships	_____	_____	_____	_____
7. Making insulting gestures, signs, or faces	_____	_____	_____	_____

Discussion among members of their responses follows.

Exercise 3. Complete the following with (a) an aggressive response, and (b) a nonassertive response.

An acquaintance has asked to borrow your car for the evening, but you have planned to use it. You say:

a. _____

_____

_____

b. _____

_____

_____

Group members share their responses and discuss them.

SESSION 2

ASSERTIVE BEHAVIOR

The aim of assertive behavior is to leave us feeling satisfied with our interactions. It allows us to express our thoughts, feelings, and beliefs in a manner that does not violate the rights of others. When you are being assertive, what message are you conveying to others? (Try to facilitate members' offering ideas similar to those given below.)

Assertive behavior says, in effect:

"I'm, O.K., you're O.K."
"I respect both myself and you."
"I expect you to respect me."

Exercise 4. Assertiveness does not mean simply being able to say no. Learn to recognize your assertive behavior. Indicate in the columns at the right how often you behave assertively in doing the following:

	Always	*Often*	*Sometimes*	*Never*
1. Saying I like, I prefer, my opinion is, I feel . . .				
2. Telling others about your abilities, interests				
3. Carrying on a conversation				
4. Giving and receiving				

	Always	*Often*	*Sometimes*	*Never*
5. Making your actions (nonverbal behavior) match your words	_____	_____	_____	_____
6. Disagreeing with others	_____	_____	_____	_____
7. Asking for directions, reasons, or to have something made clear	_____	_____	_____	_____
8. Being persistent in making requests, in disagreeing, or in standing your ground	_____	_____	_____	_____
9. Coping with criticism in a reasonably comfortable manner	_____	_____	_____	_____
10. Speaking without excusing, justifying, or apologizing for yourself	_____	_____	_____	_____
11. Knowing your rights and responsibilities and respecting them	_____	_____	_____	_____
12. Being in control of yourself, your behavior, feelings, and thoughts	_____	_____	_____	_____
13. Looking and feeling confident about yourself	_____	_____	_____	_____

Exercise 5. Complete the following example with an assertive response: You are expecting an important telephone call before six o'clock. It is now five o'clock. Someone asks you to pick up a few items from the convenience store before it closes at six o'clock.

You say _____

_____

_____

Share and discuss responses.

NONVERBAL COMPONENTS OF BEHAVIOR

Because the majority of our communication is carried out nonverbally (i.e., by what others see us do rather than by what we say), it is important to be aware of the kinds of messages we give, for example, through facial expressions and hand movements.

Exercise 6. In the exercise below, describe briefly the kind of nonverbal behavior which usually accompanies each of the three kinds of behavior labeled across the top.

	Assertive	*Nonassertive*	*Aggressive*
Eye contact			
Body posture			
Hand movements			
Facial expression			

Note: This exercise can be done individually by handing out copies of the exercise to each member, (see example below) or it can be done collectively by the members using a large chart drawn on a flip chart, blackboard, or poster. Either way, each member's contribution should be discussed by the group.

Example:

	Assertive	*Nonassertive*	*Aggressive*
Eye contact	Direct	None	Staring
Body posture	Erect	Slumped	Bent forward
Hand movements	Natural	Tentative	Pronounced
Facial expression	Friendly	Downcast	Contorted

SESSION 3

BARRIERS TO BEING ASSERTIVE

Note: First try to facilitate contributions by the group members to elicit the following five barriers and suggestions as to ways in which they affect individuals. The members can also be involved by having them write the barriers on a flip chart or blackboard.

1. *Anxiety.* We may not act assertively because of anxiety about what would happen as a result of our assertiveness. For example, we may fear hurting someone's feelings, being criticized, or even losing a friend.

2. *Guilt.* We may believe that we should always be able to please others. If we fail to do this, as for example in refusing a request, we may feel guilty. In order to avoid this feeling of guilt, we then may avoid acting assertively whenever we feel we might displease someone.

3. *Fear of feeling or looking ignorant or stupid.* We may avoid expressing our ideas assertively or asking questions because we are afraid of feeling or looking stupid.

4. *Irrational beliefs.* These beliefs, by definition, are not based on reality. They are beliefs which are not reasonable or sensible and make it difficult for us to be assertive. We develop irrational beliefs by focusing on the worst possible results and ignoring all the good possibilities of assertive behaviors. For example, "I should be perfect in everything I do." Such a belief stops one from taking chances or accepting one's mistakes. It is unrealistic to think that anyone can be perfect. To overcome these beliefs, we must challenge them and replace them with sensible, constructive ideas.

5. *Negative self-statements.* Negative self-statements are put-downs. Many of us continually put ourselves down. We say things to ourselves which are damaging to our self-respect and self-confidence (e.g., "I'm so stupid" . . . "I never do anything right"). Saying this kind of thing to ourselves and believing it keeps us from feeling good about ourselves. We are then reluctant to try new activities and miss opportunities to enjoy ourselves. It is important, therefore, to recognize our personal put-downs and to challenge them. As we change the way we think we will change the way we feel.

Exercise 7. Below are some commonly held irrational beliefs. Below each one, write a positive phrase to replace each italicized negative portion of the statement.

a. If I say what I really think, *people won't like me.*
   If I say what I really think, _____
b. If I refuse to do a favor for someone, *they will not be my friend any longer.*
   If I refuse to do a favor for someone, _____

_____

In the space below, write a few of your own irrational beliefs, and statements with which to challenge them.

_____

_____

_____

_____

Exercise 8. Write two of your personal put-downs. After each one, write a challenge or a correction of the put-down.

_____

_____

_____

_____

THE ABC OF EMOTIONS

If we follow the ABC format outlined below we can change the way we think, which will change the way we feel.

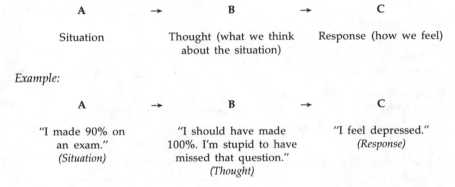

A	→	B	→	C
Situation		Thought (what we think about the situation)		Response (how we feel)

Example:

A	→	B	→	C
"I made 90% on an exam." *(Situation)*		"I should have made 100%. I'm stupid to have missed that question." *(Thought)*		"I feel depressed." *(Response)*

It is what we think or what we tell ourselves that causes us to feel depressed.

Exercise 9. Think of a situation and then think of a negative thought and response to that situation. Then replace the negative thought and response with a positive thought and the response that follows.

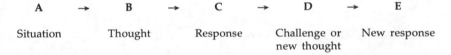

A	→	B	→	C	→	D	→	E
Situation		Thought		Response		Challenge or new thought		New response

We can challenge thoughts that leave us feeling put down and develop new thoughts that help us to maintain our self-respect and self-confidence. We will then be able to accept ourselves and react to situations in a more relaxed, less stressful way.

SESSION 4

ASSERTIVENESS RIGHTS AND RESPONSIBILITIES

The first step in learning to behave assertively is to become aware of, and eventually feel comfortable with, our assertive rights and their accompanying responsibilities.

Exercise 10. Below is a list of commonly accepted personal assertiveness rights. Read the list. Then in the column at the right, write the name of a person or situation where accepting this right would help you.

Right	*A situation or person where this right would help you*
1. I have the right to use my own judgment because I am responsible for myself.	_____
2. I have the right to be treated with respect.	_____
3. I have the right to have and express my own feelings.	_____
4. I have the right to be listened to and taken seriously.	_____
5. I have the right to set my own priorities.	_____
6. I have the right to say no without feeling guilty.	_____

Every right has one or more accompanying responsibilities. I have the right to express my opinions. The accompanying responsibility is to listen to and show respect for other people's right to express their opinions.

Exercise 11. For each right above, write one or more accompanying responsibilities.

PRINCIPLES OF ASSERTIVENESS

1. Everyone has basic personal rights.
2. We are responsible for ourselves and our behaviors.
3. We cannot change others — only ourselves.
4. If we change our behaviors so that we feel more self-respect, people will respond differently to us.
5. No one can read minds successfully. We cannot know what others are thinking or feeling unless we ask them. Attempting to do so makes for poor communication.
6. We can *learn* to be assertive.

THE DESC SCRIPT

The DESC script is described below. Use it to help plan or rehearse situations that you find difficult to handle. It will help you to avoid saying things in a self-defeating or ineffective way. DESC is formed from the key words in the four steps: Describe, Express, Specify, Consequence.

• *Step 1: Describe.* Describe to your partner the exact behaviors that are uncomfortable to you. Be as fair and clear as possible. Do not generalize or guess at people's motives. You may start with sentences like, "I would like to discuss a matter with you" or "I've noticed that..."

Example: "As I understand it, you are asking me to drive to six hockey games again this year."

• *Step 2: Express.* Say what you think and feel about the behaviors that bother you. Start your sentences with "I feel"..."I believe"..."I think..." Avoid sarcasm and emotional outbursts. The goal is to let your partner know how his behaviors affect you.

Example: "I think that is more than my share of driving. It is very costly both in gasoline and my own time.

• *Step 3: Specify.* The third step is to ask for different, clearly stated behaviors. Essentially you ask, "Please stop doing X and start doing Y instead." Best results occur when only one clearly stated request is made. Refer to changes in what your partner is *doing,* not to his personality traits or attitudes. Be prepared for the other person to make requests for changes on your part.

Example: "Please change your list so that I am called on only 3 times during the year."

• *Step 4: Consequences.* Emphasize the positive consequences that will follow if your request is met. Avoid threats or punishment if an agreement is not reached.

Example: "That way, I'll be glad to help with the driving."

Exercise 12. Use the DESC script to address the following examples:

a. A friend often telephones you late at night to talk. There is no urgency to her calls and this evening she called you at 11:35 P.M. just to chat. You have to get up early for work in the morning and would prefer she call at an earlier time.
b. You have been waiting in the grocery store line to check out our groceries. You are in a hurry and a man pushes his way in front of you saying he is in a rush and has only one item to check out.

Note: Other or additional scenarios that are appropriate for the particular members of your group might be used in place of, or in addition to, the two suggested here.

SESSION 5

BROKEN RECORD

Some people give up easily when they are opposed by others. In fact, most of us do in some situations. What we need to learn is to persist or to stick with it in saying where we stand in matters that are important to us. *Broken record* is a skill that helps us do this by repeating our position over and over without becoming rude or losing control of our behaviors.

The aim of using the broken record is to be persistent, as in Figure A-2, in holding a position in a disagreement or in making a request. The effect, after practice, is to enable you to become increasingly confident in expressing and holding your position.

Example:

Child: Mom, may I watch TV now?

Parent: No, not until your homework is done.

Child: But the cartoons are on!

Figure A-2. Broken record technique.

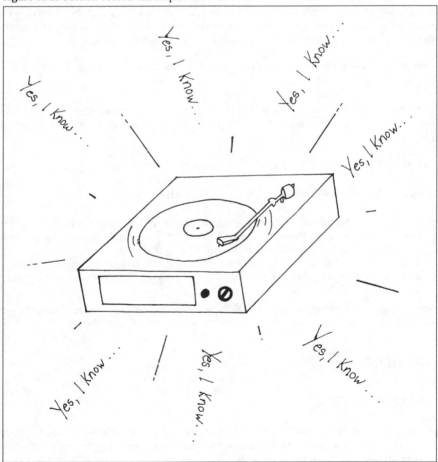

Parent: I know you like to watch cartoons, but no, not until your homework is done.

Child: You never let me watch what I want!

Parent: I know that you want to watch TV, but no, not until your homework is done.

WORKABLE COMPROMISE

Sometimes it is neither possible nor appropriate for us to get our own way and in most situations it is possible to reach a compromise. The key point in making a compromise is to make sure that the outcome does not lessen the self-respect of either person. This does not necessarily mean that each person gets an equal division of goods or choices, or an equal amount of satisfaction.

In assertiveness training this kind of compromise is called a *workable compromise*. It is a skill by which one works out an agreement with another person without either person losing or lessening his self-respect. The aim of the workable compromise is to resolve differences in position with another person.

Example:

Alice: Betty, we agreed last month that we would each do our share of the cleaning of the apartment. For the last 3 weeks, I've done almost all of it myself. When are you going to do your part?

Betty: Yes, I know you have been doing it, but I've been terribly busy. You know the band I play in is going into the competition next week. It's really important that I practice every night and when I'm finished I'm too tired to be bothered with housework.

Alice: I know it keeps you busy, but couldn't you do some of it?

Betty: You know how important this competition is! I've got to put my practicing first. You aren't very busy are you?

Alice: That's not the point. When I do all the housework, I feel like a doormat. It isn't fair to me. I think you should do your share.

Betty: I know I should but I can't right now.

Alice: I can see that the band practice is very important to you now, but I would like to work out a compromise. I'll continue to do the cleaning until the end of the month when your competition is finished. Then you can do the work next month and I'll take it easy. How's that?

Betty: That would be fine with me. Thanks for your help.

Alice: That will suit me too. If I can count on you to do your share, I won't mind doing the extra work for the time being.

Exercise 13. Practice using the broken record technique and the workable compromise on the following examples:

1. *Broken record.* You are out shopping for a blouse. You have decided you want a blue one. The salesperson insists you choose a green blouse, saying, "You look much better in green. Take my word for it, get green."

2. *Workable compromise.* You feel you are overloaded at work and your boss asks you to take on the organization of the office Christmas party. You would enjoy doing this more than some of your other responsibilities, but you know your other duties will not get done properly.

3. *Broken record.* You are asked out on a date by a man you are not attracted to. He persists in trying to persuade you to date him.

4. *Workable compromise.* You accept an invitation to attend a party on Saturday night assuming you will have the use of the family car. On Friday, your son informs you he has made a date for Saturday night and needs the car.

Note: Make up other scenarios that are suitable to the needs and problems of your group members.

SESSION 6

BUILDING SELF-RESPECT

One of the ways by which we can build up our self-respect is to take time to identify our good qualities (Figure A-3).

Exercise 14. Write a list of ten qualities you like in yourself. Think of as many areas as you can — skills, abilities, talents, habits, characteristics, values, beliefs,

Figure A-3. Building self-respect.

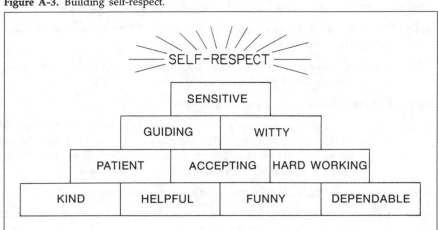

appreciation of music, art, literature, nature. Begin each statement with, "I like the fact that I . . ." (e.g., "I like the fact that I am trying to become a more assertive person"). Keep your list handy and add to it when you think of other good qualities. Read it over whenever you feel discouraged about yourself.

COPING WITH CRITICISM

There are two kinds of criticism — factual and manipulative. In factual criticism, the critic is pointing out that we have made a mistake or that the critic objects to something in our behaviors. For example, the critic might say, "You are often late for work." In the second kind of criticism, the critic's goal is to manipulate or control us by trying to make us change in some way. The criticism is not directed at the correction of a real fault or error, but having us do what the critic would like us to do. For example, "If you won't go to the movie with me, you are really inconsiderate."

Many of us have difficulty coping with errors we make in everyday life and the subsequent criticism we may receive. The criticism may cause us to feel anxious or guilty. We may become defensive, deny the truth in the criticism, attack, or try to please the critic. We can learn skills which will help us to cope with criticism in an assertive way.

Negative Assertion

The skill used to deal with criticism of a real fault or error is called *negative assertion.* It involves:

1. Acknowledging our fault or error
2. Apologizing once
3. Acknowledging the effect of our action on the critic, that is, the critic's hurt or hostile feelings or the importance of our fault or error to him or her.
4. Making amends, if possible

Example A:

Mr. Jones: Look at this letter, Jean. We can't send it out. You spelled Mr. Smythe's name incorrectly.

Jean: Oh, I see that I did. I'm sorry. I'll correct it immediately. I know Mr. Smythe is an important customer.

Example B:

Mary: Anne, you promised to drive me home from work yesterday and you didn't turn up. I was late getting home and then missed my appointment.

Anne: I completely forgot! I'm sorry Mary. No wonder you're angry. Is there anything I can do to make it better?

Negative Inquiry

One skill used to deal with manipulative criticism is called *negative inquiry*. It involves asking clarifying questions in order to prompt the critic to be direct, for example, "What is it about what I'm doing that bothers you?" Having the issue clearly defined in an open manner increases the probability of finding a solution to the situation.

Example:

Ann: Joe, you shouldn't spend so much time working on that car; every Saturday afternoon!

Joe: But I like to work on the car. What makes you think I spend too much time on it?

Ann: Well, you are always tired by the time you finish.

Joe: I don't understand. What is it about my getting tired that bothers you?

Ann: Well, when you are tired we never go out in the evening, and I like to go out on Saturday night.

Fogging

Another skill used to deal with manipulative or controlling criticism is called *fogging*. This skill is helpful when we are having difficulty saying what we really want to say, because we are feeling angry, guilty, or anxious.

Fogging involves not resisting, but agreeing with:

1. The criticism, in principle
2. Any possible truth in the criticism
3. The odds that the criticism is true while still deciding yourself what your behavior will be.

Example:

Mother: Mary, you really must make out a schedule for doing housework, and follow it. As it is, you are never caught up.

Daughter: A schedule might help me to get caught up.

Mother: Following a schedule is the best way to manage a house.

Daughter: You could be right, it may be the best way.

Mother: If you followed a schedule you wouldn't have to do the laundry on Saturday.

Daughter: You are probably right — I wouldn't have to do the laundry on Saturday if I followed a schedule.

Mother: And you should give the children the same kind of schedule I used to make out for you.

Daughter: Perhaps I should give the children schedules.

Note: Think of situations appropriate for your group members and have them suggest others where criticism has been an issue for them. Then, through role playing, the members can practice the coping skills just presented in dealing with the situations. Indeed role playing is especially useful in practicing assertive techniques (McFall & Marston, 1970) and could be used very productively throughout all six sessions.

BOOKS USED IN THIS PROGRAM

Alberti, R. E., & Emmons, M. L. (1974). *Your perfect right; A guide to assertive behavior* (2nd ed.). San Luis Obispo, CA: Impact.

Alberti, R. E., & Emmons, M. L. (1975). *Stand up, speak out, talk back!* New York: Pocket Books.

Baer, J. (1976). *How to be an assertive (not aggressive) woman in life, in love, and on the job.* New York: New American Library.

Bower, S. A., & Bower, G. H. (1976). *Asserting yourself: A practical guide for positive change.* Boston: Addison-Wesley.

Fensterhein, H., & Baer, J. (1975). *Don't say yes when you want to say no; How assertiveness training can change your life.* New York: Dell Publishing.

McFall, R. M., & Marston, A. R. (1970). An experimental investigation of behavior rehearsal in assertive training. *Journal of Abnormal Psychology, 76,* 295–303.

Appendix B
Small Group Program

Theme: Awareness of self

Sessions: Six

Recommendations:

For these problem areas:

1. Poor self-awareness
2. Lack of insight
3. Difficulty in recognizing and differentiating feelings
4. Difficulty in expressing feelings
5. Social isolation

For clients who:

1. Have a functional literacy level
2. Have verbal skills to participate in discussion
3. Are new to treatment

Objectives:

1. To provide opportunity to experience and express feelings, ideas, and opinions in a safe environment
2. To provide opportunity where giving and receiving feedback is encouraged among peers
3. To develop an understanding of oneself as an individual and in relation to others, that is, how certain behaviors affect others
4. To help individuals increase their awareness of others, the outside world, and what goes on around them
5. To sensitize the individual to the needs of others
6. To provide an environment for increasing self- and social esteem and confidence

Effective Aids:

1. Scissors and glue
2. Colored pencils, regular pencils

3. Newsprint, Bristol board
4. Magazines
5. Paper bags

Activities:

Session 1: Magazine picture collage
Session 2: How I see myself now; how I would like to see myself in the future
Session 3: Life-line drawing
Session 4: The shield
Session 5: Where am I?
Session 6: Social atom

SESSION 1

MAGAZINE PICTURE COLLAGE

Materials and Equipment

1. Large round table and chairs or space to work in a circle on the floor
2. Sheets of paper approximately 15- × 20-in., one for each person
3. Scissors
4. Glue
5. Wide selection of magazines

Procedure

The activity is introduced to the group as an exercise in which the members of the group will get to know one another through pictures. The leader-therapist should join in by making her own collage. Figure B-1 illustrates two types of collages: "Places That Would Interest Me," and "Important People In My Life."

Group members are instructed to find pictures in the magazines that illustrate the various aspects of their personality and life style. It is suggested that they look for pictures that show their interests, attitudes, likes, dislikes, characteristics, family, friends, job, feelings, ambitions, problems, etc.*

Group members could be given about 15 minutes to look for and cut out the pictures, then perhaps another 5 minutes to glue them onto their piece of paper. It is best to clean up and set aside the magazines, so they will not be distractions during the remainder of the group.

Members are then asked to share their collages with the group. Suggest that they explain why they chose the different pictures and what each represents for them. Encourage members to inquire about pictures they do not understand and comment on those aspects they see as similar to their own. Monitor the time to be sure that each member has an opportunity to share his or her collage.

---

* Remocker, A. J., & Storch, E. T. (1979). *Action speaks louder. A handbook of nonverbal techniques* (2nd ed.). Edinburgh: Churchill Livingstone.

220

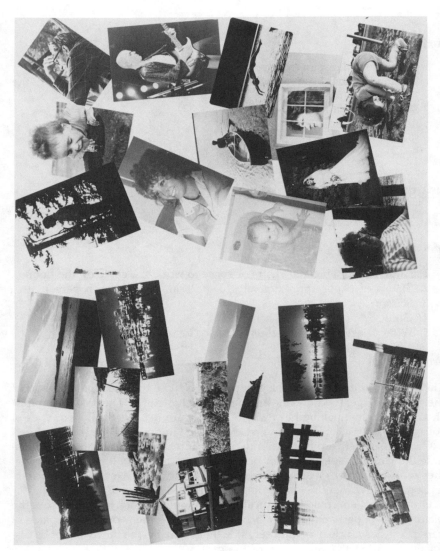

Figure B-1. Collages: Places and people.

Discussion Topics

How are members similar? How are they different? Are there any trends in the collages? Any aspects of themselves they would like to share but of which they were unable to find appropriate pictures? What are the positives and negatives in the pictures?

SESSION 2

HOW I SEE MYSELF NOW; HOW I WOULD LIKE TO SEE MYSELF IN THE FUTURE

Materials and Equipment

1. Large round table and chairs
2. White paper
3. Pencils with erasers
4. Felt pens

Procedure

While folding your piece of paper in half invite the group members to do the same. Then instruct the members to draw, on the left side of their paper, pictures, diagrams, or symbols to portray how they see themselves today (see Figure B-2 for a sample). Then, when finished with this, instruct them to draw, on the right side of the paper, how they would like to be in the future. Emphasize that artistic ability is unimportant in this exercise. Suggest that 20 minutes will probably be enough time to do both drawings. Be flexible and give a few more minutes if needed.

Ask the members to keep their papers folded and share only the pictures on the left side with the group first. When all have shared, encourage the members to find common parts or aspects of themselves. Then ask members to share the picture(s) on the right side of their papers showing how they would like to be.

Discussion Topics

What can I change? How can I change? The need to assume responsibility for making changes. Fear of changing and fear of the future.

SESSION 3

LIFE-LINE DRAWING

Materials and Equipment

1. Large round table and chairs
2. White paper

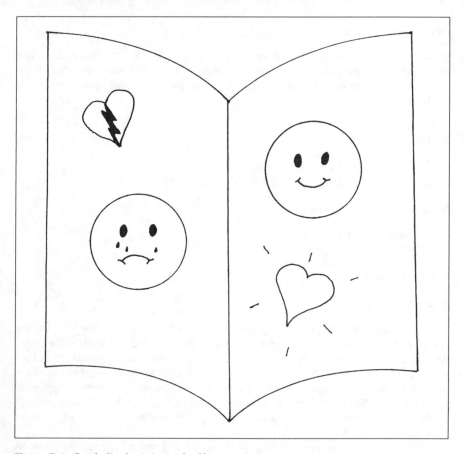

Figure B-2. Symbolic depictions of self-perceptions.

3. Pencils with erasers
4. Colored pencils

Procedure

Ask members to position their papers lengthwise in front of them and then say something like, "Today we are going to draw our life lines. We'll start at the left edge of our paper and progressing across the paper to the right, we will draw pictures or symbols representing important — both sad and happy — events in our lives. Think back over your past and try to arrange the events in chronological order. So think of your childhood first and any significant things you remember about it and then your teen years and so on." Suggest that members take 15 to 20 minutes to draw their life lines. When completed (Figure B-3 presents an example), invite members to share their drawings with the group. Encourage members to ask for explanations and to share similar experiences.

223

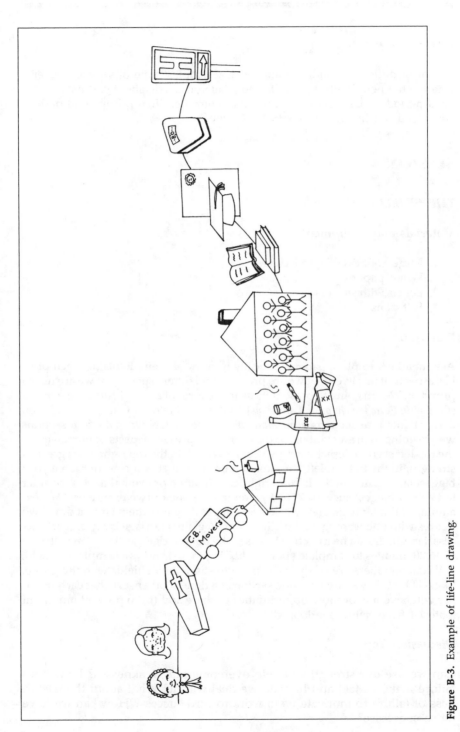

Figure B-3. Example of life-line drawing.

Discussion Topics

The most difficult period of your life. The happiest time of your life. Events where other people affect your life and what you can do about it. What precipitated periods when you felt in control of your life. What precipitated periods when you felt helpless to control your life.

SESSION 4

THE SHIELD

Materials and Equipment

1. Large round table and chairs
2. White paper
3. Pencil with erasers
4. Felt pens

Procedure

Ask members to place papers vertically in front of them. Explain, "Each of us has aspects of our lives that we are proud of and other aspects that we are not so proud of. We are going to present these in the form of a shield [*show drawing of a shield to indicate the shape and divisions*] so draw a shield on your page and then divide it into four sections [*wait while members do this*]. Now, in the four sections we are going to draw symbols or diagrams to represent aspects of ourselves. In the top left section depict your greatest weakness; in the top right, your greatest strength; in the bottom left, the situation or event that you consider to be your biggest failure; and in the bottom right, the situation or event that you consider to be your biggest success." Then go on to give one or two examples: "For example, if I think my greatest weakness is depending on others I might draw two figures with one leaning on the other, or if I feel my marriage is my biggest success, I might draw a heart or two hearts in the bottom right section. You will have 15 to 20 minutes to complete your shield." Figure B-4 shows a completed shield.

When members are ready invite them to share their shields with the group. Suggest that they share only one section at a time to (a) ensure that each member will have one or more opportunities to share and (b) to prevent important material from being overlooked or lost.

Discussion Topics

Can we use our strengths to help overcome our weaknesses? How does failure make us feel and how do we deal with it? What about the usefulness of failure to motivate us to work toward success? How can we have more successes?

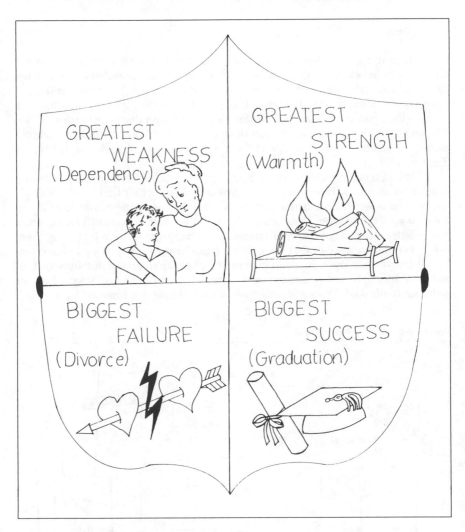

Figure B-4. Sample shield.

SESSION 5

WHERE AM I?

Materials and Equipment

1. Straight-backed chairs
2. Signs with different attributes written on them such as: assertiveness, patience, self-confidence, empathy, flexibility, humor
3. Two signs with "highest" written on one and "lowest" on the other

Procedure

Explain to the group that the exercise is designed to help them begin to see themselves in relationship to others. Ask all the group members to stand up, and then say, "I'm going to move my chair out of the group for now and leave this space. On the chair to the left of the space I'll put the sign that says 'highest' and on the chair over here to the right I'll put this sign that says 'lowest.' Then I'll put a sign on the floor in the middle of the circle with an attribute or personality trait written on it." (A depiction of what this would look like is seen in Figure B-5.)

"Think of this attribute as you progress around the circle, from very little of it (the chair that says 'lowest'), to a great deal of it (the chair that says 'highest'). You are to select the chair that represents the degree of the attribute that you believe yourself to have. If someone else is in the chair or wants the same chair you want, then you have to try to negotiate a change with them by telling them why you believe you should have that particular position. If they believe you and think you are right they will give up the position to you. If not, they will remain in the chair and you may have to try other negotiations. No pushing or shoving is allowed." You will judge when each exercise is finished by asking if

Figure B-5. How assertive am I?

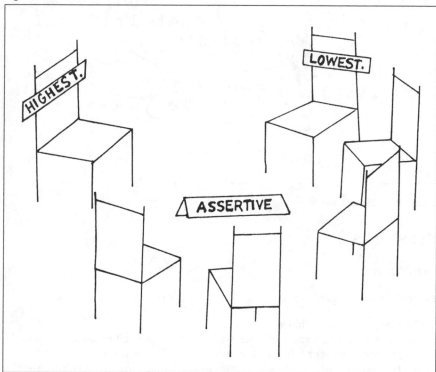

all members are satisfied with their positions. Have those members who are not satisfied try to negotiate for the positions they want. When the first exercise is finished pull your chair into the space to rejoin the circle and ask the other members to share how they are feeling and how the exercise went for them.

When you feel the discussion on that attribute is exhausted, ask the members to put the next sign with a new attribute printed on it on the floor in the middle of the circle. Again withdraw yourself and direct the members to repeat the exercise based on the new attribute.

Discussion Topics

Does the position that each member chose reflect their participation in the group? Would you like more or less of the attribute? Does the degree of this attribute that you have affect your life style, work, or relationships?

SESSION 6

SOCIAL ATOM

Materials and Equipment

1. Round table and chairs
2. Several pieces of paper for each member
3. Pencils with erasers

Procedure

Explain that each of us exists within a network of collective social atoms. The number and content of collectives varies from person to person. Some collectives are more important than others. Also, the importance of the same collective may differ between individuals. An example of what a collective of social atoms might look like is illustrated in Figure B-6.

You might say to the group, "Take about 5 minutes to draw the network of collective social atoms that make up your world. Now on a second piece of paper redraw your network and place each collective in a position, relative to your 'self,' that represents the importance of that relationship to you. Do not consider whether the relationship is important to the other party, or whether it is a productive relationship. Only consider its significance to you. To be sure the relative importance is clear, you might want to assign a number to each collective." Member X's actual network is shown in Figure B-7.

Invite members to share and explain their networks to the group. If there is time left after each member has shared and the discussion seems complete, ask members to make another drawing of what would be for them an ideal network. Suggest they diagram the types of groups they would like to have plus names or fantasy names of people they would like included. Ask them to place

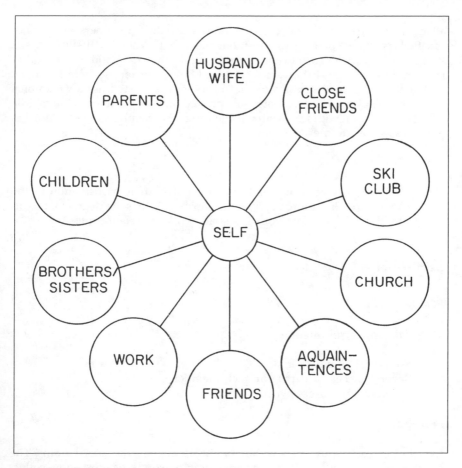

Figure B-6. Collective of social atoms.

and number the collectives as before to indicate the importance they would like the relationship to have. Member X's ideal network is depicted in Figure B-8.

Discussion Topics

Discuss the number of collectives, the number of relationships within each, and the quality of the relationships. Evaluate the collectives for vacancies, unfinished business, honest relationships, and those under strain. Which collectives would you like to add, enlarge, or diminish? Is it possible to make such changes? How would you do it?

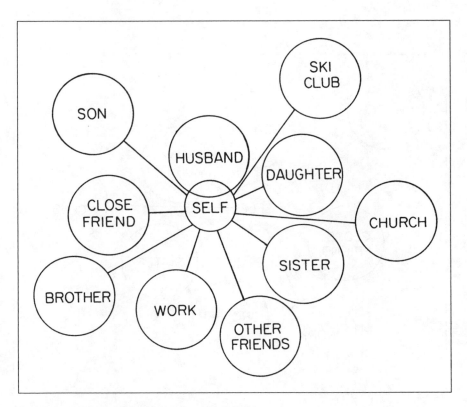

Figure B-7. Network of social atoms for client X.

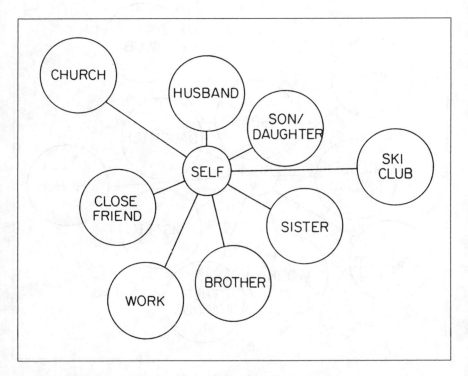

Figure B-8. Ideal network of social atoms for client X.

Index